Leukaemia - My Marathon for Love

Richard Woolley

authorHOUSE

AuthorHouse™ UK Ltd.
500 Avebury Boulevard
Central Milton Keynes, MK9 2BE
www.authorhouse.co.uk
Phone: 08001974150

First published by AuthorHouse   01/27/2011

ISBN: 978-1-4567-7423-3 (sc)
ISBN: 978-1-4567-7424-0 (e-b)

Contents

Introduction

I have a five-inch scar on my chest, right hand side, pointing towards my heart. I look at it every day and it tells me who I am.

If you are looking at this book wondering what it's about, allow me to tell you. It's about one man's experience of leukaemia and all the fun and games that go with it. It is, more broadly, a book about life and a book about death. But greater still, this is a love story. A story about how true love cannot be destroyed by things as trivial as cancer and death. Some that remember me may do so in terms of my disease. That is to say, it will be the first thing they think of when they think of me and that I was taken so young. But the leukaemia that took me was not the defining force in my life, nor was it the strongest. That will always be love, and if I do say so myself, how we managed to get it so right in the brevity of our time together. If you've read this far without vomiting, well done; it doesn't get any worse.

Dedication

This book is dedicated to Mary, Richard's guardian angel.

Background

It was April 2008, Richard was approaching his 26th birthday – yet the unexpected thunderbolt of Acute Myeloid Leukaemia beckoned.

He was always a cheerful, happy and loveable child and had successfully carried this into adulthood. Everyone who knew him loved his personality and his sparkling wit.

Richard grew up playing all sports and was particularly good at football. He achieved good exam results at school in GCSE and A levels. As to a career, he had no real thoughts other than he had an interest and real aptitude for writing. This was proven when for two consecutive years he won awards at the Chesterfield New Playwrights Competition. His winning plays were put on by professional actors to great acclaim in which he demonstrated a depth of observation in life and relationships within a comic backdrop, despite being just a teenager.

Journalism became the chosen profession and in 2004 he undertook intensive post-graduate training courses in Portsmouth. He achieved fantastic results and this really became a passionate career choice. He simply loved to write.

He met Mary when he was 17 and it was clear they were meant for each other. Their bond grew and shone out like a beacon of love to all. Their wedding date, September 12 2008, was to be the coming together of this special love and was being looked forward to by friends and family alike.

Richard was always in good health and stayed remarkably fit, sometimes without having to do much. During 2008 his weight began to drop a little which was unheard of; his colouring became ever paler, it became difficult for him to shake off any minor bugs, and his energy levels were not as good as before. Thankfully Mary, a nurse, insisted Richard went for a blood test at the doctors.

The same day, the NHS was mobilised into tracking him down and getting him into hospital as a matter of real urgency. Incredibly, Mary was at work that day in the very ward that Richard would be initially admitted to; she overheard staff saying Richard's name and that he was being tracked down as an emergency due to the diagnosis of leukaemia. The shock was obviously immense.

To help the reader, Richard's key family is made up of Mike and Marion (father and wife); Sally (Richard's Mother and Mike's ex-wife); Emma (Richard's sister) and her partner, Dave; Ben (Marion's son from her former marriage). Mary's key family consists of Ann and John (parents); Helen and Seb (sister and husband); and Michael (brother).

What follows in this book, are the notes kept by Richard in a journal, either written at the time or very shortly afterwards, recording what life is really like in the mind of a leukaemia patient; and his own words are used throughout. The dates used in the diary, also reflect the day number within the course of leukaemia, and whether chemo is being administered that day, e.g. Course 2: Day 3: Chemo Day 3; and so on. This will become clear later in the book.

The names of medical staff and patients have been changed to preserve anonymity. Family member names are not changed.

As Richard says, this is a love story, and their love will remain forever.

Chemotherapy Course 1

My Journal

Course 1: Wednesday April 23 2008

We were all prepared for the worst, the four of us who sat in my side room at the hospital, waiting for the diagnosis. In my mind I had come to terms with the fact that I almost certainly had chronic leukaemia. In a way, Mary over-hearing that snap diagnosis when she had, had helped us to get to that point. A day earlier Dr. Strong had asked me "What I'd been told." I said I knew the L word was in the equation. She nodded and moved on. My limited understanding of leukaemia at this point stretched to there being varieties of the disease classed as chronic or acute. Connotations of the word "chronic" when I first heard the term in the panic-stricken first moments of all of this, made me believe this would be the worst of the two. But when friends and family began researching, they reported that this was in fact the more mild disorder. I remember overhearing Mary talking to one of her friends on the phone, who was also a nurse, about the possibilities, and heard the friend say "At least it's not acute."

When the diagnosis came, Dr. Strong breaking the news in the best way it is possible to do, shattered us all. The words "acute myeloid leukaemia" plunged my confidence to the depths. She confirmed this was very serious and life-threatening. I couldn't look in the eyes of my family, doing so would make me cry and I was trying to prop others up with a show of strength. I said something like, "Right. Okay." I heard someone asking questions, though mentally I had drifted off somewhere very dark I do not wish to return to. Dr. Strong was explaining the difference between chronic and acute, in that acute was curable, correctable with chemotherapy, whereas chronic would be something that would remain ongoing but could be treated. Dr. Strong then began talking about choices for treatment, which I couldn't concentrate on enough to understand. Mary and Marion contained most of their tears but again, I couldn't watch them cry. Dr. Strong spent an hour talking to us and answering questions. After she left, my dad and Marion exited also, to pass on the news to other immediate family. Mary and I reassured each other. I kept a lid on things, but I think only by detaching from them. I watched a man and his two young boys laughing as they crossed the car park below my window. And I longed for a return to the time when little things seemed important.

Thursday April 24 2008

Sometimes I would wake up and forget where I was. Then it would all sink back in. Today I was to have a Hickman line put in – a tube which goes through my chest and into the pulmonary vein near the heart. It is through this that I would receive chemotherapy drugs, but it would also allow doctors easy access to my blood without the need for more needles. The Hickman line will be a fixture for a few months I am told, and something that will have to be regularly flushed to ward off infection, which I will be increasingly susceptible to as time progresses.

A doctor talks to me about the process, which is done under x-ray by a specialist whom he describes as "very slick, very quick". The doctor warns me that I will have to take great care not to catch the line on anything, particularly in the first week or so, before the skin has healed around it. He told me few common ways in which patients had wrenched out their Hickman lines in the past, including catching the tube on their belt when they leaned over, or in the lining of a t-shirt as they undressed. Knowing how clumsy I was, it was a worry. I only wanted to have one put in once.

Everyone was putting a brave face on things. Friends were telling me individually that others in their number "had taken it hard", but I never saw evidence of this. I was only ever surrounded by smiling faces and positive words. But I could piece together that some were venting their feelings while alone, just as I was. The reaction of loved ones when the news came was extraordinary. I was bombarded with cards and books, gadgets to entertain myself, and most crucially of all, love and encouragement beyond measure. Dozens of people said they would like to be tested for a bone marrow match, which is about the most humbling thing I can think of. I was feeling quite positive about my treatment and was eager to get started, but in some ways the hardest thing to deal with was how fantastic everyone was being. People kept telling me that I was brave, but at any hour of the day I never felt like tears would be far away if I allowed them out.

My dad and Marion cancelled their holiday to America which was a blow to me. Other friends talked about dropping out of a day's paintballing, which had been arranged weeks earlier, because of my absence. The last thing I wanted was for anyone to put their life on hold on my account and I encouraged everybody to carry on as normally as possible. I began to feel guilty that my dad and Marion, and Helen and Seb, seemed to visit me daily for hours at a time. People would often text me to ask if it was ok to visit, and I would tell them I was doing okay and they didn't need to keep coming in. But come in they did, because they wanted to. I tried to put myself in their position and knew I would do the same. But I still didn't want to put anybody out or trouble anyone; I'd always tried to lead a quiet life in that respect. Everyone would ask if there was anything I needed and for the most part, there wasn't – I was getting by okay. I soon learned it was almost as well to request something, small, anything. People desperately wanted to help and would leave deflated if they could not.

Though my dad had earlier begged me not to, I was trying my best to manage the feelings of everyone else, by being extra bubbly in front of those I knew needed to see me that way, or filtering the updates I gave to certain others. My dad had instructed me to think only of myself and my recovery, something I felt incapable of doing. He had already set the ball rolling on keeping my finances afloat, and had been in touch with my boss to get the lowdown on my sickness pay. He had also told Mary and me not to worry about our mortgage, which we were merely a year into, as between everyone, it would be paid – and Mary's dad had said the same. My mum offered some of her redundancy money too.

A South African doctor was the specialist who would fit my Hickman line. He was being shadowed on the procedure by another doctor, who had not seen one done before. This meant I was privy to a running commentary of proceedings and what angle to take to avoid puncturing a lung. I nervously asked how long the procedure would take, to which he replied: "My record is eight minutes." I told him I hoped he was not going for any records. I was really nervous by this point. My legs were shaking and a nurse asked me if I was cold. I could hear instruments being placed on to the tray to my right, but I was told to face away. The nurse had earlier asked me on which side I wanted the line, telling me it shouldn't cause me any real impediment either way. I felt this was a little like being asked which foot I would rather be shot in. I felt too worn out to make a decision, and said something stupid like: "Which do you recommend?" Her expression made it clear I was going to have to choose so I opted for the right side, for no other reason than that was the side of my bed where the drip machine was stationed in my room.

The doctor checked out my veins with the ultrasound machine, pointing out what was artery, vessel and bone, to the other doctor. He said I had good veins and the procedure should be no problem. He added that it was very rare that they should encounter a problem and have to open up the other side instead. First he administered the anaesthetic, Lignacaine, into the top of my chest, just under the collarbone. After little more than a few seconds, he poked the area with something and asked if it felt sharp. I told him it did not and so he made a 1cm incision with a scalpel. I know this because he was telling his associate every detail. He repeated the process near the middle of my chest, about 5 cms from my nipple, but on this occasion opened up a blood vessel. "Oops" he said, explaining to the other doctor that this was inevitable sometimes. He pressed down on the wound for about ten minutes until it had stopped bleeding. This was uncomfortable to say the least. "I don't think you're going to beat your record today" I said. When the bleeding had stopped he slid the tube down and out of the lower hole. This was pretty uncomfortable, and the doctor kept instructing me to raise my right shoulder, though this served little benefit. By the time it came to stitch up the wounds the anaesthetic had worn off, due to the time spent waiting for the bleeding to stop. I had to grin and bear four stitches in the top cut and one in the lower one. By the time I was told we were done, I felt exhausted – though the procedure had probably taken only 15 minutes or so. The grim nature of it, there was quite a lot of blood, had knocked me back a bit. The doctor and his staff wished me good luck with my treatment and I was asked to shuffle back across to a bed from the operating table to be wheeled back to my room.

En route I kept catching sight of myself in mirrors and the cold reality of what was ahead began to dawn for the first time. I had remained buoyant up to now, largely because, I think I was still in relatively good health. The shock of the surgery made me feel weak and defenceless and after getting back alone in my room I was in tears immediately. I resisted the urge to phone Mary straight away, because I wanted to maintain the perception that all was well. But my phone rang immediately, and I just ended up blurting everything out to her. She was angry that the doctor had nicked a vessel but was also upset that I was in pain. Within a couple of minutes she had calmed me down and I managed to pull myself together. For several hours after the surgery, one of the cuts was weeping blood and a number of dressings had to be put on. I was given some platelets intravenously, which helped the blood to clot, as well as some liquid antibiotics to prevent the wound getting infected. For the whole time of the bleeding my visitors, Mary, my dad and Marion, saw me suffering for the first time. I was quiet and the occasional smiles I forced were fooling no-one. After a meal and a rest, I lifted again, meaning everyone felt happy. The last thing I wanted was to see those closest to me afraid. That I couldn't handle.

During the day our wedding co-ordinator telephoned, oblivious and, probably regretted asking "Are you OK?" I told her the situation but stressed that as far as we were concerned, the wedding was still on. We needed that focus. But for now I was trying not to get worked up about going to Sheffield the following day. It was at this point I realised that the Hickman line might impede me when the time came, being as I am "right handed" as it were. I cursed myself for not considering it before. But it was too late now; I was just going to have to soldier on. Dr. Strong said my blood test for HIV, Hepatitis, etc. had come back negative, so I had a green light to give a sperm sample. It occurred to me that I had had a blood transfusion since providing the blood sample, meaning there was a remote chance I had actually contracted something since the test. Of course, there was no way I would be confessing to a blood transfusion, even if they asked me. It would probably mean another blood test and a wait of another couple of days, which I could ill-afford, as I needed to start chemotherapy as soon as possible.

April 25 2008. Course 1: Day 1: Chemo Day 1.

I awoke to the sound of one of the patients with dementia singing *Delilah*. It made a change from the *hokey-cokey* which was the sound track to yesterday. Dr. Strong came in early on to check I was in good enough health to make the journey to the Royal Hallamshire Hospital. I was told we would be travelling by taxi rather than ambulance. Ward Sister Alison talked to me about the chemotherapy I would receive, which was likely to begin that night, that being the first, then the third and then a fifth day as part of a ten day course of chemo. I knew however that further bone marrow tests would be necessary in time. Alison briefed me on the chemo, saying it may, at first, feel an anti-climax because with drugs to head off nausea, I may not feel very different at all, at least at first. I was warned to expect pink urine, however, a consequence of the colouring of one of the drugs, Daunoribicin. I was told that I could expect hair loss, which I had of course anticipated. Dr. Strong had spoken to me about it briefly and said wigs could be arranged if I so wish. I considered requesting a big blond one, just for a change, but said I would make do with a hat if I felt self-conscious which Dr. Strong recommended saying the treatment would make me extra sensitive to sunlight.

In the morning before my appointment at Sheffield, I was keen to have a canula removed from my right arm which was superfluous now I had the Hickman line in. I didn't want staff at the Hallamshire to see it and ask questions about transfusions. The right side of my chest was sore and movement in my arm was limited following the previous day's surgery but I hoped I wouldn't be hindered by it too much. I was beginning to feel the nerves now. If the chemo did leave me infertile, all my hopes of having children in the future rested on today. Mary and I had talked about having kids a lot in the past and we would both be devastated if we couldn't have our own.

Normally, when a man gives a sperm sample for IVF, he is asked to give three, at different times of the day (on different occasions) in order to get the best hope of a high count. I would not have this luxury. One chance was all I would have. My sample would then be split into three, which sounded like an awful job for someone. I began to worry that my count might be lower because I hadn't done the deed for over a week, or worse still, I may just be infertile to begin with. I tried to put these thoughts to the back of my mind, because I had to concentrate on the job in hand (whoa, mind the pun).

Wayne came to fetch me for the taxi and we got on okay. I wondered what there would possibly be to talk about on such an excursion. He asked me about how I was diagnosed and what life was like 'before', suggesting, as I already suspected, that I would view my life either as one before, or after, leukaemia. It would be my year zero. I told him that before, things felt a little monotonous. Don't get me wrong, I had a fiancée I loved more than anything, a wedding to look forward to, I'd even just started a new job. But despite all this it was like something was missing. The only way I can describe it is as if I was waiting for something life-changing to happen. I told Wayne that just maybe this was it. The people who are most full of life are often those who have flirted with death, as though they have been galvanised with verve for living. I felt that if I could just get through this, I'd be so much closer to those around me and everything would mean more. As warped as it sounds, I hoped I could look back on this as a blessing.

When we arrived at the Jessop Wing of the Hallamshire, I had managed to channel my nerves into determination. I was called into the Andrology Dept. and taken through a series of forms setting out what would happen to the sample, and any subsequent embryos, should I die. The general gist was that my sample would be stored for 10 years, after which time the decision to keep or destroy it would be made between the parties concerned. The Co-ordinator (tall, bald, seemed to smile all the time) explained that my sample would be analysed to determine its quality, before being frozen, providing it passed whatever quality control they applied. In a few weeks time a small portion of it would be de-frosted to see how well it had reacted to the freezing process. While we were going through all this, it was difficult to take my eyes off the sample pot on the desk in front of us. I had wondered what it would look like. If you are curious, it was clear plastic, about 2" tall and tapered so it was, slightly wider at the top with a screw lid. I was ushered into a side room, back past Wayne who glanced up from a magazine. I could hardly lock the door quickly enough behind me. There was a treatment table inside, a chair and a sink. Then there was a table scattered with various literature. How much detail do you want? Suffice it to say I got to work. Minutes after I was shown in, I heard a bloke being led to the room next door. Less than 5 minutes later, he was off. I wondered how long it was customary to take in these situations given there was no-one to impress. There wasn't really anyone I could ask now. I looked at the variety of magazines and wondered how much the NHS spent on pornography each year, and whose job it was to buy it. When I had finished, I got dressed quickly suspecting time was of the essence with my sample. I placed the pot inside the bag I had been given, curiously marked "Biohazard", washed my hands, and walked out of the room.

By now there were several men in the waiting room, none of whom could resist glancing at the bag. I put it on the counter as I had been instructed and caught the eye of Wayne, who had dealt with the embarrassment of the day rather well. He gave me the subtlest of nods and said "Let's go". While we were waiting for the elevator, I saw Wayne clock the fact that my belt was still undone. A rather graphic oversight on my part. We had a wait of around half an hour for our taxi, during which we watched the buzzing of crowds of people coming in and out of the hospital. A man who was dressed like a doctor answered his mobile, his ring tone being the theme music from *Scrubs*. I thought how the surreal nature of today's events would not be out of place in that show.

On the ride back to the hospital we hardly spoke, mainly because the radio was on quite loud, but also because I was no longer having to take my mind off the nerves. I felt pleased that now I had given us a chance of having children where otherwise it may not have been possible. I was grateful to Dr. Strong for arranging the appointment so quickly, when she had not been fully behind my decision. Now I was keen to begin the chemotherapy. Dr. Strong had earlier explained that the cancerous cells are increasing by the day, thus raising the level of leukaemia in my body. We couldn't afford to waste any time and back at the hospital Dr. Cowdrey told me he wanted the treatment to begin that night, which I was grateful for. Over the course of the day several people came to see me, and we all had a good laugh at the day's events.

Later I was hooked up to the first chemo treatment via my Hickman line. I was already becoming more accustomed to the tube that was protruding from my chest. Yesterday it had felt very alien indeed. I couldn't lie flat because I could feel the tube pressing on the side of the vein, so had slept last night propped up at 45 degrees. But it was still far from being a part of me. The main discomfort, other than the paralysing terror of accidentally ripping it out, was the feeling like something was stuck in my throat, which no number of gulps could dislodge. This was not a constant niggle, however, and for the most part I could live with it being there. It was still a watershed moment when they connected the first bag of Daunoribicin (red one) no matter how eager I was to get started. Mary watched the drugs go in, and kept saying under her breath "I can't believe this is really happening".

A couple of my friends kept telling me I had become a minor celebrity of *Facebook*, the social networking website, though I disputed this. I had no way of keeping track of my profile, but was assured that well-wishers had been leaving messages of encouragement through my page, or Mary's. For those not familiar with the site, one function allows the user to add a status update telling their on-line friends what they are up to. This can range from the funny to the surreal to the mundane. I often liked to just put a song lyric up there, I remembered that the most recent one I had posted, and therefore one that would be there for a few weeks yet, was quite fitting. A snatched line from my favourite Bob Dylan song, it read *Let me forget about today until tomorrow*.

Saturday April 26 2008. Course 1: Day 2: Chemo Day 2.

It was hard to believe I had only been in hospital for one week. So much had happened and my life and that of those closest to me, had turned on their heads. The night before I was admitted, I had been at the pub quiz with friends, joking around. That seemed like someone else's life. Ideally I could have done with more sleep but such a commodity was difficult to come by on Durrant Ward. I would notice others on my ward, who were almost entirely elderly, would spend a lot of the day snoozing, whereas I was always awake from 7 a.m. until midnight. It was starting to catch up with me a little, but the constant coming and going of nursing staff, housekeeping, caterers, the occasional doctor and my constant relay of visitors, made it pretty much impossible for me to get any meaningful sleep during the day. But at night, some of the patients really came alive. The nurses would often tell me how short-staffed they were on nights, and I felt sorry for them when I heard two or three buzzers going off at once. The previous night an elderly man had 'opened his bowels' as the nurse had put it, outside my door. There was a patient toilet near to the entrance of my room but for whatever reason this man had not made it that far. From what I could gather, as I lay on my side in the darkness of my room, he was spreading the mess around with his foot. He kept repeating to the nurse, who was trying to make him stand still, that he "wasn't bleeding". Episodes like this were not uncommon, but nonetheless had an effect on everyone on the ward, it certainly did on me. The impact must have been far greater on the elderly people packed into the bays, separated by gender, and the noise must have been much worse than for me in my big private room out of the way, right at the end of the hall. Other patients would often size me up as I passed, and I wondered if I was being judged. Why did this young lad, who is upwardly mobile and seemingly in fine health, have his own room. Or maybe they knew why.

By this time I was on several medications, as well as regular paracetamol. I had tablets to ward off gout and fungal infections, which people with leukaemia are susceptible to, and I was given a dose of antibiotics twice a day to boost my immune system. Also given twice a day were anti-sickness tablets, designed to negate the effects of the chemo drugs. Then there was the mouth-wash. I was to gargle four times a day, which got a little tiresome, but it was necessary to keep the risk of infections at bay. On the positive side, my teeth had never looked so white.

The days were, to my surprise, flying by. I think this was because they were divided into so many parts. I would be woken for monitoring observations, pulse, blood pressure and temperature, at 7 a.m. Breakfast was at 8 a.m., chemo treatment at 10 a.m., some more observations, then perhaps one of the doctors would stop by, dinner at 12, choosing tomorrow's meals, visitors, more visitors, maybe a little walk down to the hospital shop, more observations, tea at 5 p.m., more visitors, some time alone with Mary, a second chemo treatment at 10 p.m. etc.

People had brought me countless books and things to amuse myself with, but I had hardly touched any of them. My room was already cluttered with a mass of gifts and some visitors would attempt to tidy up but just ended up moving things around so the clutter was slightly re-ordered.

The chemo treatment was rather daunting at first. The pharmacy would send up a self-contained pack, made up of all the various things needed, including the drugs themselves, saline, gloves and little vials of a sterilising liquid. The nozzles on my Hickman line would be wiped clean, before a saline drip would be hung above my bed. The clamp on the Hickman line would be released, allowing the flow to begin. The feeling of a cold solution being fed directly to the heart is a strange one, something I felt I would never get used to. The chemo drug, Cytarabine is then fed into the solution via a valve on the saline wire, using a syringe. The saline is allowed to run for another couple of minutes or so to flush out the line. It is then disconnected. That's it for 12 hours. Daunoribicin was slightly different in that it was fed by a drip over the course of an hour, but I only received this drug on days 1, 3 and 5 of a ten day therapy process. It did, as doctors had warned me, turned my urine a fetching shade of pink.

Now a couple of days into the therapy, I was waiting to be hit by the effects, almost craving them, to reassure me the drugs were working. So far I had felt just a little woozy now and again, similar to a mild travel sickness. Staff kept telling me the affects could yet be several days away. Perhaps I would regret yearning for them when the time came.

Sunday April 27 2008. Course 1: Day 3: Chemo Day 3.

I made a couple of attempts to steal some sleep after breakfast, but staff, visitors and the throb of the ward made it impossible. I had the dose of Daunoribicin in the morning along with the Cytarabine which I received twice daily. Gavin warned me that the red one was often the one that made people feel more ill. He told me about patients in the past, who thought they could take the drug as it went in, often causing them to retch. Thankfully I did not have this problem, although I was still nervous before every treatment. I didn't want this to be happening. I didn't want to get ill, or for my hair to fall out. Most of that afternoon was plagued by nausea. Mary was bringing in bits of food to supplement what the hospital was giving me, but my stomach was turning. The thought of eating anything made me want to vomit. Marion suggested I tried eating little and often, but this was even more unappealing. I preferred, if I had to eat, to have a full meal and so not to have to tackle anything else for 4 hours. Even drinking water was unpalatable, and taking all my pills took several minutes sometimes, to ensure I didn't see them again. It was a bit like a bad hang-over, one that now looked like lasting for a few weeks. But I knew things would get much worse before they got better.

The chart I had been given didn't spell out how long the third and fourth courses of chemo treatments would take. This we were keen to know, as we had begun looking at the calendar and trying to ascertain where our wedding day would fit into the whole process, preferably at the end of it. Of course, there was no way to be exact. A lot depended on how quickly my body bounced back after each bout of chemo. The drugs would kill the cancerous cells but also the good cells in my blood. Dr. Strong had likened it to putting weed killer all over a flower bed. It might take 3 to 4 weeks for the average leukaemia patient's blood to begin bouncing back. But as Dr. Strong pointed out, I had youth on my side. It might take me only 2 to 3 weeks. The gruelling aspect of chemotherapy, however, is that as soon as you begin to recover and feel better, they hit you with the next round and put you back on the canvas. Ideally a patient will go into remission after the first round of chemotherapy, but even if they do, they have at least another 3 rounds of treatment to look forward to. The theory being that just because the harmful cells are not visible, it doesn't mean they are no longer there.

Best practice is to frazzle them completely with at least a 4-round salvo. There is a chance I could yet be randomly selected for a fifth course (20% of the people on the trial) something it was not known whether there was any benefit to. But while I had my eyes firmly locked on the destination, there was the chance that my chromosome tests might reveal me to be 'poor risk' meaning other treatments would have to be considered. Likewise, if I didn't respond to the first 2 bouts of chemo by going into remission the same would apply. All this was weighing on my mind and I didn't know whether it was better getting ahead of myself and picturing myself healthy at the end, or just to take every day as I found it. I settled on somewhere in between.

My nausea hadn't settled by the evening and a nurse provided me with some of those charming cardboard vomit trays. I made a grab for them a couple of times, but didn't need to use them in the end. I didn't know if these were some of the first outward signs of becoming ill, or just a reaction to the drugs.

One of the signs that something had been wrong prior to all of this and prompted Mary to order me to have blood tests was that I'd lost weight. Despite being tall, I have always been slight. When I was healthy I had weighed just under 11 stones, but that had fluctuated to as low as 10st.6lbs, just recently. I could always eat anything I liked and never put on weight, so to lose half a stone was distinctly odd. Mary, who was on a mission to lose a few pounds for the wedding, was annoyed that I had dropped so much weight without even trying. Now in hospital, I was weighed once a week, in a wheelchair with a calibrated seat. Gavin had panicked me when, doing a quick 'guestimate' in his head after weighing me in kilograms, he reckoned I was about 10 stones. I made an involuntary gulping sound, genuinely worried. "That can't be right" I told him. He checked the conversation chart and reported it was actually around 10st.8lbs.

Monday April 28 2008. Course 1: Day 4: Chemo Day 4.

I began to feel really lethargic and weak. We went for a walk down to reception and I felt like I was floating along the ground. I felt the chemo start to bite and I went right off my food. I managed to force down a little bit of dinner at 12.00 but was fighting nausea all afternoon. It was a little like having a hangover though I always want loads to eat when I am nursing one. When my tea was brought in I vomited. The sight of the jacket potato flipped my stomach, which was odd because the potato at dinner was the only thing I felt safe eating. I felt better afterwards, but my tea was sent back untouched.

We had been playing cards to take my mind off the sickness but it got through in the end. I was placed on another anti-sickness drug, on top of the one I was already receiving and was even given a dose intravenously to settle my stomach. While this took the edge off it the nausea did not go away. I knew more blood transfusions would be a possibility and I hoped they would help because all I wanted to do at that moment was sleep all day.

Later that evening, my temperature started to rise. A tell-tale sign that I might be coming down with an infection. The nurses kept an eye on it. They tried to take a blood sample from each arm but left with nothing because they couldn't find a vein.

Tuesday April 29 2008. Course 1: Day 5: Chemo Day 5.

I woke feeling very ill. On top of this my back was really hurting. I didn't know if this was a symptom of anything or just the fact that I'd been lying down for so long each day. I had suffered from back aches since I was in primary school, just as my dad had. He told me he always feared I would suffer the same lower back problems he had, which had culminated in three of his vertebrae having to be fused together. He would have felt responsible if I had. I got the impression he probably felt in some small way responsible for my leukaemia, as ludicrous as it sounds, even though the doctors told us it was nothing more than a genetic fluke.

Over the course of the day my back-ache escalated into easily the worst I had ever had. I couldn't get comfortable at all, but was far too weak to try to walk it off. My temperature had continued to climb steadily, hitting as high as 38 degrees. This confirmed I had picked up an infection which was probably in its early stages. Despite my temperature being high I felt very cold and shivery. My first instinct was to cover up with a blanket, but this only served to inflate my temperature further. Mary instructed me to take off all my covers; she pointed an electric fan on me and placed cold flannels on my forehead. Needless to say, this was difficult to stand. My temperature stopped rising but remained in the ballpark of 38 degrees, somewhere around 36 degrees being normal. I was given doses of IV antibiotics to fight the infection and Dr. Cowdrey, the other consultant, put me on a small dose of steroid to help combat the sickness. I had vomited again that morning and, though I recognised eating was important for my recovery, I just couldn't face anything. Dr. Cowdrey was concerned enough to give me the steroid, which he had earlier confessed a reluctance to prescribe. I needed to stop vomiting if my chemo was to work at its best. I was told to keep drinking lots of water, which I had less of a problem with. Just like yesterday all my body wanted to do was sleep, and I actually dozed off for a couple of hours while Mary, my dad and Marion were visiting. It was now painfully clear I would not always be able to put a brave face on things, despite my best intentions. I felt very ill indeed and was quite withdrawn and uncommunicative.

I was scheduled for 3 units of blood to boost my immune system, which had improved my health and palour the last time I had received it, several days ago. I was now on what felt like dozens of drugs and potions, which would be laid out before me in little plastic cups over the course of the day. I actually nearly choked on one of them that morning after casually tossing it into my mouth. It went down the wrong way and I had to drop on all fours and make comedy barking noises to hawk it back up. I was grateful nobody had witnessed that embarrassing little episode.

I was beginning to exhibit some of the other side-effects I had been told to expect, such as a sore mouth and constipation. While these were no big deal in themselves, on top of everything else they didn't help. I was feeling a little sorry for myself, which is not like me, but

10

it was getting increasingly hard to smile. This had been the worst day so far by some distance, and there was no way for me to tell how much worse things would get. A friend visited me at around lunch time and must have left with a warped view of how I was doing. I didn't want to let her leave having seen me at my lowest so far, and reporting back to others that I was at death's door. But, in the end, I just had no fight in me to convince her otherwise. I tried to crack the odd joke but for the most part we sat in, more or less, silence. She watched me pick at my dinner before sending most of it back. It's difficult for some people to know what to say. I was gutted that she had left having seen that. It was much the same for Seb, who came in that night to watch Man. Utd. beat Barcelona in the Champions League Semi-Final on the little portable TV. By this time I was feeling a little healthier but was in agony with my back, so didn't talk much during the game.

In the night I woke up and my sheets and pillows were completely soaked. At first I thought I had wet the bed, but soon realised I had been sweating profusely. My temperature had still been high before I turned in, so I was being monitored for it through the night. Despite feeling freezing cold, I was sleeping with the fan on and just a sheet to cover me. During the night this served to break the fever and at around 4 a.m. my temperature reading was actually lower than normal, meaning I could now cover up to get warm again. My sheets and pillow cases had to be changed, however, as they were soaked through.

Wednesday April 30 2008. Course 1: Day 6: Chemo Day 6.

By comparison to the previous day I was doing cartwheels today. It felt fantastic to have broken through the despair of yesterday. I felt that, if these peaks and troughs were going to be the norm, I needed to make the most of the good days. I was determined to do more when they came round. I wanted to get outside to stretch out my aching legs and back. I wanted to demonstrate I could bounce back. I had a shower and got dressed. Today could be a normal day. I was getting more au fait with my medical procedures and the multitude of drugs I was taking. The doctors told me I would become an expert on my condition in time, and noticed I was picking up more and more nuggets of information each day.

As I dressed I could hear a man down the ward shouting "I need a friend, I need a friend", which stopped me in my tracks. I could hear one of the nursing staff soothing him in a lowered voice, but couldn't imagine what they were saying in reply. His words kept cropping up in my head over the course of the day, lodged in there like the lyrics of a pop song, and I would mull over the sadness of it. Here was I being showered with gifts, cards, and encouraging words when others around me seemed so starkly alone. It just made the generosity and love of everyone around me feel that little bit harder to carry. Everyone likes to be the centre of attention for a little while, but to be thrust into the spotlight and become the centre of several peoples' universe, is, I found, more than a little embarrassing but I owed everyone so much, and if all I could do to reward them at that moment was to show them I was doing okay, then that was what I would do.

I made sure I was in a chair when my visitors arrived, to demonstrate I was up and about. It was an instant boost, to them and me, for them to see me back on form. Mary especially was lifted by it, and I drew all the positive vibes I could from her smile. I remember telling her she was "the best" and she repeated the same to me. I joked "I know. Hardly seems fair on everyone else that we're together." The rest of the day, as it turned out, was a rather foolish show of bravado on my part, and I ended up wearing myself out. By the evening, my health had plummeted again. I felt colder than I ever had, despite my temperature going back up to 38.8 degrees. The relatively sleepless night was a sign that I needed to change my attitude a little. I couldn't attempt to carry everyone's feelings.

I could sense I was becoming weaker by the day. My world was shrinking, and it had to afford me the best chance of getting through this. I had all the time in the world to ponder every aspect of my life, but I could go days without thinking about some of the things I previously drew comfort, satisfaction or pleasure from. I already knew this experience would change me for the better.

Thursday May 1 2008. Course 1: Day 7: Chemo Day 7.

A bad day. Spent most of it dozing on the bed unable to get up. I couldn't even communicate. This was getting tough. Temperature shooting all the time. Visitors from Portsmouth, managed half an hour with them before going very tired and temperature spiking. Mary having to do everything for me. Felt as weak as a new-born, utterly helpless. Worst day yet. Starting to get me down, realise this is going to be much harder than expected. At night, I noticed blood in stools, very sore.

Friday May 2 2008. Course 1: Day 8: Chemo Day 8.

Lots of bleeding from my back passage. Very painful and very worrying. Dr. Griffiths, chubby, bland, doctor bloke, gives me rectal exam. I am given extra medication for the pain including small dose of morphine. This helps a bit but I am at first unable to pass water and they discuss putting in a catheter. Eventually I go though. Later on I become really hot, unusual as have been feeling cold all the time. Tried to cool down in a cold shower and have a kind of fit called rigor. Am crying out and shaking involuntarily unable to snap out of it. Mary comforts me but is terrified. Doctors say I just need to ride it out. It lasts more than 45 minutes and I eventually pass out into sleep. Most scared I have ever been.

Earlier in the day we get the news that my sister Emma isn't a stem cell match. What we expected and something we hopefully wouldn't need anyway. Despite this Emma was upset as it would have been a way for her to help very directly.

Saturday May 3 2008. Course 1: Day 9: Chemo Day 9.

Staying positive but all the effects are really mounting up. I am on two different mouth washes but my gums are red raw, which makes it a real chore to eat anything. I haven't slept continually for a period of more than an hour for four days. I haven't eaten a proper meal for a week. I have to dash to the toilet every hour for a very painful toilet ceremony. My temperature constantly fluctuates between normal, high and very high. All this combines to make me feel extremely weak.

Emma visits, at a low point, and I can hardly look at her let alone hold a catch-up session. The rest of the day is very up and down but I feel I hit the bottom, but worse was to come when I had a reaction to some of the drugs, which I suspect was the strong pain-killer Servidol. I had already had two small doses during the day and another one in the evening. Soon afterwards I felt like someone had injected rocket fuel into my brain. I became more wired and alert than I'd ever thought possible. My chest went hard like wood. It felt like my heart was pumping overtime. I was vividly aware of every sound and smell around me. I was beginning to panic and spoke briefly to Mary on the phone. Fifteen minutes later, despite it being late, my dad arrived to help get me through it. Just having someone around made the tough spots easier. He sat with me for hours as I panted, scratched, and scanned the room with my eyes. When it did eventually clear, it felt like my head had shrunk to half its normal size. For those three days where I thought I had hit the bottom, I still went deeper.

It's hard to even think clearly now. People have to repeat things and I miss words out when I write things down. I lose sentences near the beginning and trail off. I feel I am having the moisture sucked out very slowly by the tiniest straw, and all that's left is a teacup in the desert. I receive two units of blood.

Sunday May 4 2008. Course 1: Day 10: Chemo Day 10.

Night most disturbed so far. Hallucinating when I close my eyes, but don't even realise this is what is happening. I am aware there seems to be separate realities running around me, I just hadn't got round to naming them yet. My temperature is very high. I question things quietly, and remember something Dr. Strong saying about being able to opt out of having treatment at any time. Not left these two rooms in four days. I wait for the hands to tick into daytime because the humming in my head is better when the lights are off. I try to remember at what times I have my observations and medicines, but can't. Out of nowhere, mercifully, I begin to pick up as it gets lighter. But I am watching every minute go by until 2 p.m. Something changes from then. I come back to life. The ever-changing cocktail of medicines makes a break-through and my health lifts considerably. It feels as though I'm allowed to have a crack at a puzzle on a new day, having previously attempted it blindfolded and drunk. My mood surges, there is work to be done when the sun shines. I shower properly, I have conversations in a style other folk do as I might have once. I eat food. Don't get me wrong, I cannot lift a car or walk the length of a hallway even, but I am dizzy with euphoria. I felt I had been ground down so low I wouldn't come back, now I was determined to fill this void with something solid, so when I came this way again, I would be of sterner stuff. The cancer had made its first mistake.

Monday – Thursday: May 5 – 8 2008. Course 1: Days 11 – 14.

Various adventures in health. Get outside in the wheelchair a few times. My wheelchair only goes backwards though and being seated hurts my arse. It has made trips to the toilet a real lottery but I will not accept any of the doctors' painkillers after the side-effects of the last one, I'd rather be in pain.

Beginning to dread the nights. The place becomes very haunting. I've been hardly sleeping and when I do it is a very light trance, just below the surface and then only for an hour at a time. I begin to learn that 10 p.m. chemo treatments or drips can be hours late by the time the nurses get round. This is just one of those things with staffing what it is around here, as far as I can learn from Mary anyway. But there is an unsettling air after dark and the nights seem to last for ever. In one of my trances during one of them, I'd managed to convince myself that two nights had passed, so long did it last. My temperature had now held level for over 24 hours, much to the delight of the doctors, who had scratched their heads over the various antibiotics I had been given and why nothing could seem to get it under control. I was finding it hard to feel anything about anything. All I felt was tired and washed out. Nurses would try and pass the time of day with me, but I was so utterly exhausted at times it was all I could do to smile and agree. It was already far tougher than I had imagined it could be and my personality had been dumped unceremoniously on the back seat while my survival instinct, or whatever was left of me, took the wheel.

I learned by this point that some of Mary's family had started an appeal raising cash for the two of us, to give us something to look forward to on the other side. The 'appeal' would be known as *The Woolley Hat Fund* and the main event would be on F.A. Cup Final day. I didn't know if I would be well enough to attend although I suspected not.

The ward had filled up with women all at once, who Gavin assured me, were harder to look after and more demanding. No surprises there. There were some old boys who were characters though. I overheard a nurse asking one of the men where he was from. "Pilsley" came the reply. "Ooh, very nice" she said. After a barely noticeable pause he said "It's not, it wants a bomb on it".

Friday May 9 2008. Course 1: Day 15.

My night was very disturbed again and I'm functioning on very little sleep. I worry I'm not eating or drinking enough and resolve to try harder. Going to the toilet is still very painful and a couple of times I rethink the painkiller option. The pain is impacting on my quality of life, making me feel apprehensive about going and perhaps even putting me off eating more. Then again, I cannot handle the thought of any repeat of the effects from last time. I decide I may discuss it with Dr. Strong, but I'm not going to chase the issue.

I receive some platelets early on in the day, to help with clotting ahead of them taking out my stitches. One had already been removed days earlier, but an angry-looking blood blister put the nurse off tugging at the other one. In the end it came out with a little more persuasion and didn't bleed at all.

Boredom was, by now, getting to be a common enemy. The days were no longer flying by as they had to begin with. They were now a real slog. Filling the hours from early morning to when my visitors got here at 2 p.m. was the biggest job. I had DVDs, CDs and books around me, but with my brain working flat out on what was going wrong in my body, it was difficult to draw any pleasure out of any of them.

It was really just a waiting game, which I do not like to play. Knowing I had to go on in this current routine for another two weeks made me feel sick. Before, the regime had been changing and things were new to me. Now I wasn't even on the course of drugs anymore, just sitting around all day, day after day, waiting. I found it grim, because all I wanted to do was blitz through the treatment and get well, but it wasn't the way the game worked. As a consequence of all of this, I was getting short-tempered. I hadn't snapped at anyone, that's not my style, but I wanted to at times. I caught myself complaining a fair bit to family and tried to rein myself in from doing it so much. To tell the truth though, I was very unhappy, it was difficult not to be really. I missed everyone, I missed my life, I was so tired and so utterly bored of being in pain all the time that smiling had pretty much dropped off my daily routine. Little things were beginning to grate on me. The drip machine in my room was very temperamental and would always stop a couple of times during blood transfusions and make an awful noise. Every time it did I would glare at it with pure hatred. On this one occasion it kept breaking down and the idea of smashing the thing to bits, spraying blood everywhere, filled me with lust. The cheap alcohol hand-wash smell was getting on my nerves. The daylight hours buzz of the construction site outside my window was annoying. The intermittent signal on my TV would just drop out when it felt like it. I was tired of being cold all the time to keep from spiking a temperature. All of these things were minor and I knew it, but there was some small comfort to be gained by venting frustration at something.

Saturday & Sunday: May 10 & 11 2008. Course 1: Days 16 & 17.

I decided to accept a sleeping tablet to help my body catch up on some sleep. In the night I woke and dashed to the toilet and was in agony afterwards. I couldn't be a hero anymore and begged for one of the pain killers. Over the next couple of days I had a few of them and found them to be actually quite enjoyable. They gave me a nice drowsy, relaxing feeling and I was happy it seemed they had found something I could get along with. After a day or two, though, I began to break out in a rash of red spots, that looked like an allergic reaction or some sort of heat rash. The doctor examined me on the Saturday, uttering the words I was becoming all too used to: that the relevant specialist/department was not available over the weekend. This had been the case when I first came in on a Friday night, and other complications which seemed to evidence themselves at the weekend. It puzzled me slightly that specialisms and departments took weekends off, when illnesses and disorders did not, but it was just one of those things. By now I was becoming increasingly downhearted at how my health could yo-yo. I would find myself deteriorating in a very short space of time, often just minutes. My temperature would shoot up and I would feel weak, tired, ill and just withdrawn into myself. I was beginning to notice patterns during the day such as always taking a nosedive during the early evening.

Others were enjoying some warm weather, but I hadn't felt well enough to go out for the past couple of days. It had been suggested it may just be a heat rash, I hoped so, but expected it to be a reaction to the pain killers and to be taken off them. I felt like I was falling apart. My hair was coming out slowly but surely, I was covered in red spots and my lips had swelled up. I had looked better, in short. I was taken off some of the liquid antibiotics, which Dr. Woodward suspected was behind the reaction but warned that a) it may take 3 or 4 days to notice any benefit, and b) I may not notice any benefit at all since it may not have been responsible for the rash at all. "It's a process of elimination and we'll continue as we are" he said. My rash was by now a scattering of angry red spots which covered my legs, arms, stomach and feet, making me look like some kind of X-file. My eyes were also sore this morning and dry round the edges, I seemed to be collecting side ailments by the day and wondered how many more I could be asked to reasonably endure.

In the wider world, it was the last day of the Premiership football season. I watched all the scores play out on *Ceefax*, each permutation bringing agony or ecstasy for one set of fans. It had been a nail-biting season which had come down to the last game with the champions, places in Europe and two relegation victims to be decided. My team, Portsmouth, were to appear in the F.A. Cup Final next weekend and ever since getting through a month previously, had looked intent on losing every game. It did not bode well for a final in which we should have been runaway favourites. My chances of going to the final had been well and truly torpedoed. Mary's family had arranged a big fund raising event in our honour for F.A. Cup Final day, and I'd heard on the grape vine that a few football clubs had been contacted with a view to donating auction items and raffle prizes. I thought the chances of me being able to attend were very low indeed, it would have been too much of a stretch health-wise, too busy and I would have been worried about getting to toilets and things. All that was assuming I would actually be well enough, which was a long shot to say the least.

I thought about other milestones on the horizon, king among which was of course our wedding. The venue seemed to be quite flexible with dates, and would allow us to change without cost. That was nice to know, but as far as I was concerned 12 September was our wedding date and I was going to be well for it, come what may. Mary had said it was just a date, and if we had to move it a week or two then so be it, but I felt the date was within reach.

Monday May 12 2008. Course 1: Day 18.

My temperature and health was still up and down all the time, but, though it was varied, the way I was feeling was way below feeling human, feeling myself. It felt like such a long time since I had been me, and I just couldn't see an end to it all. I felt like in some small way, I had died several deaths in my mind but had yet to be reborn. I was in a very dark place in my mind. People were telling me I needed to ride it out and stay brave but I just didn't feel that I could. I was running on empty. My hair had been dropping out in little strands over the last couple of days but it hadn't had an unnoticeable effect on the way I looked. I sat in bed for some time looking out the window, then very calmly got a carrier bag and began running my fingers through my hair, sometimes quite roughly, so it began to come out. It came in strands or it came in clumps, but it was coming out, and I continued for what must have been a couple of hours until around half of it was gone. Large portions of my scalp were now visible and the rest of my hair, usually very coarse, was now thin. I asked Mary to bring in some hair clippers to shave the rest off. I just wanted it gone; I wanted something, anything to change. I wanted a watershed moment. Maybe I just wanted to look the part, I don't know.

By today my rash was an angry purple mess and was the most unsightly thing I had ever seen on my body. It had spread onto my stomach, chest and even face, though it was by far the worse on the lower body. I had a talk with Dr. Cowdrey, who looked through my drug chart and asked why I was having no pain relief, other than paracetamol, which is the painkiller of choice for those who like pissing in the wind. He put me on regular doses of a painkiller I'd dabbled with over the first couple of days, which by now I was all too happy to agree to. He also put me on a light steroid to help with the rash and my itching, sore eyes, another new development. He put me on a couple of things to ease my constipation and gave me a cream for the pain down there. I was heartened by the positive steps he was taking to make my quality of life better. He had news too. My blood tests from that morning showed my haemoglobin (red cells) and platelets seemed to be holding at the levels of my transfusions a few days earlier. If this was the case, it meant that, hopefully, my white cell levels might begin to pick up as well. If they did, they could set about repairing all the various ailments I had and quickly make me feel better. It was very encouraging to hear, but I didn't want to get too far ahead of myself. I had to take every hour as it came and forget about tomorrow. Tomorrow was another century.

My health dipped again in late afternoon and I went shaky and tired. But a little later on it improved slightly and I asked Mary to shave my head. She took no pleasure in it, and seeing me looking so different was a bit of a shock to us both. But it made me feel purposeful. I felt like a Royal Marine shaved and ready for a scrap.

One other worry by now was that one of the tubes in my Hickman line was blocked. It would be clotted with blood, so could not just be flushed through into my main vein. My fear was that if they both became blocked I would have to have a whole new line, put in under the surgeon's knife. I was terrified of having to undergo that again. I was told that Alison, the Ward Sister, was something of a specialist in unclogging the lines, and that she would be informed of the blockage.

Later in the evening I started to feel healthier, then healthier still, peaking at my highest point for several days. My sense of humour had returned, and I was able to have a laugh with Mary and her brother Michael when they were here. Michael had been my only visitor outside of the core of my dad, Marion, Mary and my Mum for several days. Michael had timed it perfectly really and I remember telling him "It's nice to see a different face, even if it's yours". It had been suggested earlier that I should try and see some other friends and family occasionally, if only to bring some variety to the days, a relief to the monotony I had described. It made sense to me and I realised I had been keeping people at bay as much because I didn't want them to see me, as because I didn't feel up to seeing them.

Because I felt healthier, I hoped I might sleep better, but this didn't transpire. Again I slept very lightly, barely south of conscious at all. Here I was aware of noises and movements even though I was technically under, and though I slept more deeply for the odd hour, it was another disappointing night, that took some time to end. I was paranoid about my temperature spiking again, and felt I had lost my ability to tell if I was actually hot or cold, so I just had to aim to feel cold all the time, windows open, fan on, clothes to a minimum, even if it got uncomfortable which it often did.

Tuesday May 13 2008. Course 1: Day 19.

By now I had been given the cream to help ease the pain after I went to the toilet. It was called Anusol, which I distinctly remember laughing at the name of several years ago when I saw it advertised, not because I was feeling immature particularly, just because the makers of it had not shied away from getting in the matter-of-factness of the word "anus" in the title, thereby sparing no blushes over the pharmacy counter. I had laughed as I imagined the scenario of people whispering its name to the pharmacist, and having to repeat it several times at a barely more audible level, before probably losing their temper and just bellowing "A-NU-SOL!." Now here I was with my very own tube, albeit having obtained it the easy way. This meant two things: 1) most probably poetic justice for me for having laughed several years ago at the name, and 2) I was going to need to select a new finger for applying my mouth ulcer gel. Anyway, it helped a bit so let's say no more about it.

Today was the best I had felt in probably two weeks. I can't actually stand properly for more than a few seconds, walk distances even. This I did a little, not to make anyone feel better but simply to take advantage of being able to stretch my legs out. I chatted more, obviously, and had the odd joke, but had learned it was counter-productive to get excited and try to be my normal self, because I wouldn't be able to sustain it. I was also philosophical about these pockets of health, having learned to my cost, several times, that getting giddy about it just made the subsequent crash all the more soul destroying. I had developed this mechanical way of thinking about things, a selfish way of thinking about things, I felt, out of necessity. It goes against everything I stand for in normal life, but this was not normal life. A large number of forces were acting upon me and normal rules had long since ceased to apply.

I had also been thinking more on the fund which had been started in my name and was feeling more uncomfortable about it. This had nothing to do with pride, more to do with having a clean conscience. I felt that, if I could get out the other side of this and get healthy, it would be its own reward. I wondered if I could allow myself to take this sum of money, whatever it might be, and use it for something like a recuperative holiday, clothes, entertainment, whatever, when there were people just beginning the journey I would have made. There were charities which could help research treatment and improve lives for those undergoing them. My head was spinning over the whole thing. On the one hand I desperately wanted to do something with and for Mary, because she had been so wonderful, but knew that she would support whatever decision I made. I also didn't want to upset or offend anyone who had donated money to us, for our benefit, by giving it away. I resolved these were decisions we wouldn't have to take until much later and I may feel vastly different about things by then, so there was little point in giving it further thought now. Besides, I was feeling and looking healthier, so it was important to spend time with visitors I had kept at bay, and try and eat more. So that be wot I dun, like, all the time hoping my white cell counts were on the up.

Wednesday May 14 2008. Course 1: Day 20.

Following such a good day, it was perhaps inevitable I would come down to earth with a bump. I was now very constipated again and the discomfort was limiting my movement significantly. I discussed it with Dr. Cowdrey, who was annoyed that my drug chart showed I hadn't received any of the Senna I had been prescribed. This drug encourages the bowels to work and softens things in that area. He prescribed me a double dose for that evening with a view to getting things moving. I had, by now, become accustomed to having to talk about such personal matters with everyone, several times a day. The doctors would come in altogether every few days, or in pairs on the other days, and ask me questions about my bowel movements, how much I was eating and drinking, if I was in pain, if my mouth was still sore, and about my rash, which had settled into a browner colour but was none-the-less ugly. I would give an answer and they would buzz away among themselves, suggesting which new drugs may help and which I probably no longer needed. "Should he still be on this steroid?" "Well I hoped it would help to boost his appetite." Sometimes I couldn't hear or understand the discourse and would sit there on the bed looking from one face to another until one would smile at me and say something like: "Alright, thanks. You're doing well." Then they would all file out of the room. On this occasion, before doing just that, Dr. Cowdrey said my white cells were still showing no sign of picking up. For some reason this seemed to hit me quite hard, though I didn't really react at the time. "But," he said, "there's still plenty of time for improvement yet and we still won't be worried if that's the same situation in a week's time." I don't know why I had hoped the white cell count would have shown miraculous improvement already, I wasn't even aware I had been harbouring that expectation until Dr. Cowdrey had told me otherwise. But I felt a little bit cut up by it, as well as apprehensive since my white cells were obviously the route of my problem.

I was a little withdrawn that afternoon, partly because of the news, but also because I had been placed on a heftier dose of painkiller. It left me feeling very sedated and unable to do anything more than lie in bed in a daze. My arm was still hurting from the latest blood test that morning. The phlebotomists were usually very efficient in getting blood out of me painlessly, but this morning had been very painful indeed. The needle had felt all wrong when it went in, but then the lady proceeded to move it around inside my arm to release the blood flow. I was actually crying out that it was really painful, to which she replied "it will only take a second, darling. It's bleeding out now." It felt very alien and continued to sting for a long time after the needle came out. This was, of course, the test that revealed my continued lack of white cells, so it was especially galling to get that news when I felt my discomfort more than warranted a report of bustling white cells. But it wasn't to be and I had little option other than to go on as I had been doing – which didn't involve much of anything at all other than moping around waiting to be told "You're cured my boy! There's the door, off you pop.

Mary's cousin Sean came to visit in the evening and I sensed he must have been greeted with the stark truth of what was happening to me. There I was, bald, covered in some sort of biblical plague rash, hardly able to lift my head off the pillow because I felt so weak and sedated. I couldn't even smile properly, because of all the ulcers and lesions in my mouth. This bothered me quite a bit because smiling works both ways, as we all know.

Mary had been to her G.P. earlier in the day and reported back that he had signed her off work for another month. She didn't feel able to go out and do her job properly, with so many other things on her mind. Then there was the fact she wanted to be here for long periods every day, particularly in the evenings, which she knew were tough for me because I would get apprehensive as the dreaded nights closed in. Add to that her fear of picking up any infection, however small, from a patient she was treating, meaning she had to stay away until further notice. The G.P. was very sympathetic, and agreed to review the situation on a rolling basis. He also prescribed Diazepam, to Mary, to settle her nerves and aid sleep as and when required. It was useful to have to fall back upon, we agreed, but something which should be reached for sparingly.

In the evening I wrote out a card from myself and Mary, which I had asked her to pick up in the day, to my dad and Marion. It was just something small to thank them for all their love and support thus far, but something I hoped might lift their spirits in some small way. It was also important to me, at such uncertain times, to make sure those around me knew how important they were to me, since I wasn't comfortable expressing it fully in normal day to day life. But if I couldn't do it now, when could I?

Thursday May 15 2008. Course 1: Day 21.

The adjoining ward to Durrant, on which I was based, had been closed off for a couple of days. The ward, whilst still running behind the scenes, had been isolated after an outbreak I learned was Clostridium Difficile, or C-diff, one of the "super bugs" often depicted as a spectre over our hospitals by the media, along with MRSA etc. C-diff is a very nasty sickness and diarrhoea bug, which can be deadly to those at their most vulnerable. I heard that security measures had been stepped up after a number of cases, and a barrier now stretched across the entrance to Eastwood Ward, barring visitors and giving orders on hygiene. I was at the furthest point away from Eastwood Ward, but noticed in the morning that an infection control sign had been placed on my door, warning that it was to be left closed at all times. I would be lying if I said I was totally unperturbed by those developments, but felt secure enough in what myself and staff were doing that it wouldn't be an issue. It was difficult not to worry about infections and the like, however, it would have been foolish to be blasé about it. The fact of the matter was that I still had no immune system to speak of, other than the doses of antibiotics, and I was at risk of anything in the air or that which was usually dormant in my body, progressing into what the doctors called a 'septic episode', which I found to be a lot like feeling really ill only worse. But I wasn't about to turn into Howard Hughes. As long as I and those around me were sensible we could minimise the risks. Anything that was going to get through was going to get through, and that was that.

My weight was now around 9st.8lbs, which was quite a loss for someone with my frame. My doctors were concerned by it, as was I of course, and they kept stressing the importance of eating as much as I could. I understood this fully and couldn't get my head around why I was losing quite as much weight as I was. By this point I was making good efforts with my meals and eating all of them for the most part, and having the odd snacks in between that I could manage. I was also doing very little that could be classed as burning off calories to any significant degree, because I had been so weak of late but the effects were really starting to show. For the last few days when I'd looked in the mirror it had been to monitor my rash, but now when I looked beyond that it was clear how gaunt I was becoming. My face, neck, torso, arms and legs were all looking noticeably thin. It's easy to wonder why I didn't just sit and gorge myself and, believe me, in my previous life that was a hobby. The problems were layered. 1) I had a complete loss of appetite. Food just held zero appeal and the idea of eating just felt out of the question. 2) Eating was a real chore. By now, I could hardly open my mouth because of the ulcers, couldn't chew anything harder than a soggy pea and even swallowing hurt. 3) Nothing tasted of anything. Hardly any flavours, sweet or savoury, came through my taste buds. For my whole life I had drawn so much pleasure from food but now eating was just something wretched I kept getting ordered to do more of. I was told by the doctors that a dietician would be round to see me some time in the next couple of days, which I knew would probably result in me subscribing to the milkshake supplements I had already sampled and convinced my stomach were a good idea against its better judgement.

Friends of friends who had been through chemo treatment had offered to lend me an ear or advice about the whole process, which was really touching. It could be useful to talk to others who had been where I was and who could offer encouragement from their experiences. But I didn't know if I felt quite ready to talk to a stranger about it all. I felt I was still a long way from grasping the situation in my own mind and coming fully to terms with it. It was still all so shocking and unexpected, that if I just pondered the enormity of it during a quiet moment it would either freak me out or make me cry. Perhaps that's what I needed, but I just couldn't surrender to it. I had cried on Mary's shoulder several times, but they were all like showers rather than the dam-burst I probably needed to release. I was learning a lot about myself and the way I deal with things emotionally, and to tell the truth little of what I was learning pleased me much. I had imagined when all this began that I would be much more bullish and defiant through the low times, but when they came I found I just wasn't capable of the humour and high spirits which I always felt were the very core of me. I felt so subdued for such long periods of the day. This could be put down to a combination of my illness and the somewhat Draconian effects of all the drugs I was taking, but, though I wanted to, my personality couldn't break out and say: "Fuck you, I'm still here." It was in a glass prison below the surface, watching everything like a deaf mute. Of course, on a good day or, during a good hour, part of it was less paroled and I felt alive again. What frustrated me was how infrequently it got the chance. Even when I felt more or less okay, I behaved a bit like an automaton. But then this was life in a very small box with all the colours turned down, and perhaps it was asking a bit much of me to be bursting into song.

Friday, 16 2005. Course 2: Day 22.

I missed Mary terribly. Though she was here every day and we got some time alone it wasn't the same. I missed our lives together and the way we sparked off one another when we were at home or out for the day. We would hug and talk but it just wasn't enough. I missed, I suppose, the intimacy of what we shared. It was nothing to do with sex, since my treatment seemed to have sent all desire into hibernation. Mary missed me too and we decided to try and arrange a day that was 'just us'. I knew my dad and Marion, who had likewise been here every day, would understand the request, I was just mindful of myself being able to phrase it well enough not to cause offence. The pair of them desperately wanted to be here as much as they could but I thought they, too, would benefit from a day to themselves to recharge the batteries and think about something else. It was win-win, as long as I could keep my foot out of my mouth when explaining it. I was now 11 days post-chemo and, in theory, should be feeling better by the day as my counts recovered. One day next week could be the perfect time to do it, as obviously we'd both prefer it if I wasn't a basket case for the day. There was no way to be sure, though of course, but come hell or high water, we were going to have a perfect day even if every step of it had to be forced or engineered. A bit of planning wouldn't go amiss, I resolved, but that could be taken care of later.

All the excitement of the past weeks had really put a dampener on the fact that Portsmouth, my dad's and my team, were in the F.A. Cup Final – as favourites. It was the biggest game for us in living memory but a series of snags had lined up to push it backwards in our minds. Okay, so there was my leukaemia diagnosis first of all which was a bit of a downer in general but, that aside, the game was against Cardiff, which held little appeal for the neutral fan, therefore there was virtually no buzz around the game whatsoever. Then there was the fact that our beloved Pompey had contrived to lose their last four games of the Premiership season, which hardly inspired confidence in the fans going into such a massive game. But Goddammit here we were, in the final, and the occasion needed to be savoured. There was of course the F.A. Cup Final Party being hosted at Mary's Auntie Sheila's taking place on the Saturday afternoon, which was a fund-raiser for *The Woolley Hat Appeal*. Though nobody was quite sure of what the attendance there would be, I should probably set the scale of Sheila's parties. She is a warm and wonderful human being with a heart of gold, and strike me down if she can't throw a soiree to prove it. The family house is an imposing size and upstairs there is a huge games room with a projector and big screen, ideal for sporting events in other words. I knew no expense would be spared on drinks and catering, so everyone was in for a cracking day (and night) it was safe to say. I was just sorry I couldn't be there. It was just too soon and would have certainly been too much of a stretch for me to even pop in, since it was a fair distance from the hospital. The plan therefore was for my dad and Marion to watch the game itself with me in my room, before they headed off for the party. Now it was down to my team getting their arses in gear and making sure they brought home the cup. Tomorrow was going to be a big day.

Saturday May 17 2008. Course 1: Day 23.

I was hoping against hope for a healthy day, but woke feeling really groggy and not very well-rested at all, despite having accepted a sleeping tablet the night before. My attempts to grab a couple of hours sleep in the morning proved futile. Unusually for a weekend, there seemed a full complement of staff buzzing around, and the ward was especially noisy with the comings and goings of patients to the toilets and the sombre procession of the catering trolley.

In my daze I was administered two doses of a painkiller over the course of the morning. I had begun to question the necessity of it once again. I could sense Dr. Cowdrey was only persevering with it because he was keen that I eat enough and not be put off by the train wreck inside my mouth. But the painkiller was the last remaining thing which could be making me constipated and I was keen to remove that problem once and for all. When Dr. Cowdrey made his rounds and asked me how I was feeling, I replied that, disappointingly, I felt a lot weaker than I had the day before. My head felt stuffed to bursting point with chatter I had little control over, and I found it quickly exhausting. It put me in mind of my earlier reactions to the stronger painkillers, in which my thoughts were not entirely my own. Physical side-effects are one thing, but the ones that altered my mental state really scared me. I was being withdrawn from all the drugs day by day, and I resolved to stop the painkillers immediately. Cold turkey. After I fed back a muted response to my feeling of wellbeing to Dr. Cowdrey, he allowed himself a smile and said "Well, that's interesting", and then dropped some bombshell news. I had known for a few days that the platelet and red cell levels in my blood were climbing, but had only heard the day before that my white blood cell reading had climbed to 0.1. Today, however, it would seem my body was staging some kind of Charge of the Light Brigade. My white cells had surged and my neutrophils had reached a level of 0.2. I had barely reacted to that nugget of information when Dr. Cowdrey added: "So, depending on another blood test in the morning, there's a good chance we'll be able to send you home tomorrow." I swallowed. I felt tears begin to fill my eyes. I was so shocked I could hardly move. When I had first been diagnosed, the doctors had talked about getting me home for the odd day or two. Here, he was suggesting I bugger off until a week on Wednesday, when I would be expected to saunter back in for the formalities of a bone marrow test. Still stunned, I asked if my latest counts suggested a successful round of chemo. In response no less guarded than I expected, he replied that it certainly looked positive that the chemo had been successful and <u>may</u> have sent things into remission, but without the accuracy of the bone marrow test it was too early to speculate.

It was a heart-stopping moment in which I felt a dozen emotions collide inside me. It was so unexpected I felt rooted to the spot. I never dreamed I'd be going anywhere for over a week. Dr. Cowdrey left me with the good news, which he had obviously enjoyed imparting and I immediately phoned Mary. We both burst into tears as we talked about the simplest of comforts of being at home together, something that we had previously taken for granted. She was over the moon, so was I, but for a few niggling doubts which had begun to eat away at me. Chief among these was fear. I had been living for a month in a guinea pig cage, being constantly watched, probed and poked, fed with drugs and remedies, etc., etc. For all the mental torture of that, it felt safe. The idea of leaving hospital early was a frightening feeling. Had I become institutionalised already? The comfort of being surrounded by doctors and a team of nurses was pretty much what I wanted when I was wallowing in the ditches of health. I confessed my fear to Mary, who as a qualified nurse, would be dedicated to my case around the clock, and could easily have taken offence. But she did not, and reassured me the hospital would stock us up w........................ they would discharge me. Nevertheless, this good news weighed heavy on my mind all day, and my health began to plummet.

I managed barely a few spoonfuls of my dinner before collapsing into bed, cursing myself for feeling so weak again on this, the day of the game. I began to suspect I was withdrawing from all of the drugs they had stopped giving me over the last couple of days. I was now down to a couple of tablets a day, and had consciously decided to abandon the painkillers.

The Match was a bit of a blur to me. I was watching it but not capable of digesting everything that was going on. Nobody was expecting a classic, but it was pretty dull. Portsmouth took the lead through Kanu after about 35 minutes, and the rest of the match was basically the clock winding down. I began to struggle in the second half, like my body was crying out for things I couldn't give it. I felt guilty that my dad had been forced to watch the game in such circumstances. Had things been different, he would have been at the game, sharing the history of a momentous win. As it was, he watched it with me, his son, in that little room in Chesterfield Royal Hospital, on a TV with a crappy signal. But I stole a glance at him during the game and knew that, for those couple of hours, he didn't want to be anywhere else.

That evening was tough. I was receiving a flurry of text messages from people at the fund-raiser taking place at Sheila's, and I felt too spun-out mentally to respond to many of them. I was withdrawing from the painkillers and, not for the first time, having serious doubts about my sanity. I felt like I was following and observing myself, watching TV, reading or pottering to the toilet. I was hallucinating again and had no clarity of thought.

Late on I began to get worked up and got chest pains. A kind nurse, a big smiling African guy whom I hadn't met before, chatted to me to try to calm me down. He talked to me about my guitar, where I'd got it, was I any good? Was I in a band? He told me that he used to play, and was keen to start again. I took deep breaths and tried to calm down, but everything was right on top of me. The nurse told me I should have a sleeping tablet, to calm me down and let me get some rest. I snapped back that I didn't want any more drugs. I wanted to get my mind clear of everything; I wanted to get out of the tunnel. Again he recommended I take a tablet, just to calm me. It would help. I heard myself begging "No, please. No more. I can't take anything else, I won't." He was quite insistent that I should take just this one thing to calm me. It would get me through the night and in the morning everything would be different. "In the morning" he said "everything is always different." He went to get the tablet, while I stood in my room shifting from foot to foot. He returned and got me into bed, handed me the pill in a little cup and I reached for the glass of water beside my bed. I put the pill in my mouth and washed it down. One thing was for sure; it would be a tough night going it alone, and I did need some help. "Good man" the nurse said. "In the morning we will talk and things will be different." He left and I stared around my room wondering how long it would take until I felt more relaxed.

I thought about things being different tomorrow. Not just tomorrow, but later on down the line, when this was over. How would I be different? I thought about when people utter that old cliché "I'm the same person, I haven't changed." I never buy that. It's as if admitting to changing is a sign of weakness or a betrayal of self. I say we're all changing all the time. How can we not? Every experience we have gets picked up by the snowball. Every choice shapes us. And when something really significant comes along, triumphant or traumatic, it alters us.

Sometimes only those closest, those who know us best, will notice. Only a few may see the join. Or maybe no-one will. But we are never the same, even from one minute to the next. Why fight that? Why deny it? In the morning, things are always different. How this whole experience would change me I didn't know. I hoped that Mary would recognise enough of the person she loved on the other side to want to stick around. I wondered how she would change in all this, after seeing me so utterly vulnerable. I looked at a picture of her that was fixed to the mirror in my room. She is wearing a striped top on a night out. She had one finger to the side of her mouth in a gesture that is hard to describe, but it's somewhere around a tipsy, flirty look, that at some time is shy and self-conscious. She is happy. And in that moment she, is so perfect, so beautiful, that I realised that everything was going to be okay. To my right was a card she had written me just days earlier, which read "When I fell in love, I am glad it was with you." Somehow the word 'love' didn't seem to do it justice. Sometime later, though I wasn't aware of it creeping in, I went to sleep.

Sunday May 18 2008. Course 1: Day 24.

Hospital pillows are cold. I am not sure how they are different from pillows at home, but they just feel colder. Perhaps it was partly down to me getting used to being bald. I would wake up invariably in a little pool of dribble. This, I am sure, was down to the problems with my mouth, but nevertheless I would wake up stuck to a cold pillow. I was glad of the sleeping pill. Without it would have meant another largely sleepless night and I was beginning to realise just how much of an impact they were having upon me physically and mentally. The fact of the matter was that the hospital was simply not conducive to rest. The constant noise and coming and going of staff and patients would interrupt even the most modest attempt for 40 winks. Then there were the patient buzzers which, suffice it to say, were so constant they became one of those things that fade into the background. They are there but they are not there. Like the wallpaper. There was usually at least one going off within ear-shot at all times of the day and night.

All this process, treatment and recovery, was still new to me, and I was learning day by day. And the shapes of my foes were revealing themselves. It was clear the battle had two lives; health – the actual fighting of the disease and infections, the sickness; and the psychological battle – getting through this with my sanity. The two elements were fiendishly, interlinked and inseparable from one another, but there was one question which scared me the most. Poor health had been incredibly hard to deal with but it was the mental anguish of the darker moments when I felt closest to breaking.

Each morning I would tentatively sit up and try to do some sort of audit of how I was feeling. How were my energy levels? How clear was my head? Did I feel rested? Did I feel sick? It's a difficult thing to take stock of, and the shape of how I was feeling would only really reveal itself as the day unfolded. Today, however, I was especially keen to see how I would feel, as there was a chance I would be going home. I wanted to feel fighting fit, but soon realised I did not. It was not a bad day by any stretch, but, as usual of late, I just had no energy to speak of at all and I didn't feel alert in the slightest. I knew I was down for another blood test this morning, and my passage home was resting on the result. The idea of leaving hospital did scare me, but I was coming to realise the benefits would greatly outweigh that. I needed proper rest and proper food and I would get neither of those things here.

The phlebotomist took some blood from me at around 10 a.m. I looked at the clock. It was a Sunday, perhaps that would slow down the turnaround of the result, perhaps not. Either way, the early days of time flying by for me in hospital were dead and gone. The hours dug in their claws and their heels and a morning could feel like a lifetime. Filling up those hours was an art form; I felt some way off perfecting. My mind was playing tricks all the time and granting me an almost non-existent attention span. I would put on a DVD or start a book and my mind would nag at me like a spoilt child, telling me it was rubbish and questioning why I was bothering. I couldn't draw any enjoyment from anything. Days earlier, I had found a book, lent to me by my friend Paul, which managed to break through and capture my attention. I found The Kite Runner captivating and I got a release from reading it. The only problem was, I consumed it in two days and was back to square one looking for something else.

While I waited for Dr. Cowdrey, who I had been told was on his rounds, I didn't know whether to begin packing up my things or not. In a month I had amassed a great deal of stuff and the walls were covered in cards. It was going to be a big job to get it all out of there, but get it all out I must as there was no guarantee where I would be put when I came back in. When Dr. Cowdrey entered he was smiling and I sensed it was good news. I had really warmed to Dr. Cowdrey, having been unsure how to take him at first. I had found my range with him and now found him warm and approachable. Just like Dr. Strong, he carried an obvious wealth of knowledge, experience and expertise on his shoulders. I had been told by several parties that I was being looked after by the best two doctors in the hospital. Dr. Cowdrey confirmed my counts were looking good. My white cells were up to 1.3 and my neutrophils were 0.3. My platelets, he added just as an aside, seemed to have doubled overnight. I could go home.

By now I was off every medication bar an anti-fungal infection pill and the two mouth washes designed to combat infections in my mouth. I would be sent up a prescription from pharmacy that afternoon, and then I could go. My Hickman line would need to be flushed through before I went but otherwise, that was that. It was a dizzying feeling and I felt I needed to thank Dr. Cowdrey for this miracle they were performing on me. I tried to do just that and say something heart-felt, but he was packing up his things and moving on with a smile. He gave me an appointment card for that Wednesday on Cavendish Ward, when I was to come in for a blood test. Depending on what that revealed, they might go ahead and perform another bone marrow test there and then to determine what effect the chemo had had. Dr. Cowdrey hinted that if my counts were something approaching normal, they may arrange to get me back in a little earlier than planned to begin phase two. That was positive as far as I was concerned. The more time that could be shaved off the process to get me well for the wedding was a priority. I didn't just want to be present at the wedding; I wanted to be fighting fit for the best day of my life. I made the call to Mary and asked how she would feel about having me at home. She cried and seemed to like the idea. Then I told my dad and Marion who were equally keen to get me out of there. My dad, ever the resource, said; "We've got loads of boxes."

So the four of us packed up my things and I was wheeled out wearing a trilby, guitar strewn across my lap. Employing a series of diversions, each cleverer than the last, we escaped. The drive home was a surreal one. I gazed through the windscreen of my dad's car like a puppy on its first car journey. Summer had exploded on the world while I'd been sleeping, and the avenues were bathed in glorious fanfares of green. The world had been reborn in a vivid new dimension of colour. Of course, I was the only person for whom this had happened suddenly and, as such, the only one who'd noticed. My remarks about it just sort of floated away on the pollen-rich winds. I thought about all the incredible things we never notice. "In the morning everything will be different," the nurse had said, not knowing how right he was, the wise old goat.

We pulled up outside my house and I went inside as the others got together my possessions they wouldn't let me lift. I wandered from room to room, surveying the ghosts of some past life. Half-read magazines, CDs from the party we'd hosted the weekend before I went in, a worn T-shirt discarded on the bedroom chair. The clock had stopped here when I first got that phone call that woke me from some peaceful dream and shattered everything. Mary hadn't been staying here since. She had been sleeping at her Mum's each night, unwilling to pay more than flying visits to our home, which had ceased to be that for a while. But now we were here together, and that was all it took to restart the heart of the house.

Just being out was a boost but I was disappointed in myself for not feeling stronger. I wanted to feel the improvements Dr. Cowdrey assured me were taking place in my blood, but I did not. But at least the setting had changed, and that was stimulus enough for now. In the afternoon Mary and I walked to our local shop to get some essentials. Though it was only 100 yards or so away, it proved a stretch for me, and revealed just how weak I had become. I suspected that I had gone somewhere beyond malnutrition and my body was beginning to give out. Being so slight I simply didn't have the reserves to drop so much weight so quickly. But I could feel my appetite was returning and my mouth was repairing itself. That meant, I hoped, that in the coming days food was going to be making one hell of a comeback. I managed two good meals and we went to bed, our bed, which felt like the most extravagant thing in the whole world. It was insanely comfortable and warm. It was absolutely silent. As I dozed, I remember, quite involuntarily, mouthing the word "bliss".

Monday May 19 2008. Course 1: Day 25.

With the benefit of a good meal, a good night's sleep and the psychological massage of being home, I realised just how much hospital had been holding my recovery back. The main improvement had been up top, with the demons of my neuroses now silenced. I also felt worlds better physically. I was grateful for Dr. Cowdrey getting me out of there, even though I hadn't felt ready to leave. It could scarcely be a better set up, with the hospital only five minutes from where we live, and Mary, the qualified nurse, determined to wait on me with everything I needed around the clock. We laughed at that part of the arrangement, as I was conventionally the fetcher, carrier and general dogs' body in our relationship, which was only fair seeing as care was Mary's job and I wanted to spoil her and take care of all that when we were together.

To say my appetite was back didn't really do it justice, I had been overtaken by a hunger so singular of mind that I found it conceivable to simply sit and eat from sunrise to sunset. My body was in weight gain mode and we were going to need supplies. Mary got a pen and paper to make a shopping list and all the requests began tumbling from my mouth. She raised an eye brow and took it all down, before heading off to the supermarket to harvest enough calories to give the entire Olympic squad heart disease. The fridge was full. For now. The change in my eating was nothing short of comical. I would eat a bowl of cereal and then go and eat another, wash up the bowl and then decide "no, I'm going to go and eat one more." If we went out for half an hour I had to fill up my pockets with fruit pastilles.

Despite all this eating, I wasn't really feeling any stronger. I couldn't walk or stand for very long but didn't know if I would be better advised to try and rebuild some fitness or just rest. At one point during the day my phone rang upstairs and I tried to hurry upstairs to answer it. My legs buckled under me and I ended up in a heap at the top of the stairs with my legs throbbing and Mary telling me at volume exactly where I ranked on the idiot scale. But I was determined that, when I went back into hospital to face down the trauma and trials of chemo, I would be stronger. I needed to be.

Tuesday May 20 2008. Course 1: Day 26.

My nights were now a lot more restful, but still fractured. I would wake several times, soaked in sweat, needing to go to the toilet. The nights would also see my mental demons return. I felt as though I was watching myself, sometimes from very far away, and operating remotely. My thoughts felt crowded with my brain's involuntary chatter about subjects which were sometimes relevant but usually not. One night I was trying to let go and sleep, but couldn't switch off for my brain twittering on about origami, the subject about which I knew nothing. I would get a song, seemingly picked at random from everything I'd ever heard, stuck in my head, and my brain would kindly play it for me, the parts I knew anyhow, over and over and over again. I had no control over any of this and began to fear for my sanity again. What was causing it I didn't know. I was now free from all my medication apart from an anti-fungal infection tablet so it couldn't be put down to a side-effect of anything I was taking. My fear was that the stress and sensory deprivation of my mouth in hospital had done me lasting damage.

Physically I was still very weak. Walking even short distances was dizzying. Mary and I walked out to a little card shop on our road and I had to lean on her most of the way. We took it slowly but when we got home I collapsed on the sofa and slept for an hour. I couldn't picture being normal ever again. The energy levels required to go and do a day's work were so far beyond what I felt capable of at that point that I just couldn't imagine ever getting back there. I was a fit and healthy 25 year old man just a few short months ago, now I was reduced to this. I broke down a couple of times during the day, just because I felt so helpless. Mary was finding it hard to keep a lid on her emotions as well. Though she was my full time carer, confidante and guardian angel, she too felt helpless and it was hard for her to see me failing to cope.

We both had the worry of tomorrow's hospital appointment hanging over us. I was due for a routine blood test for an up to date measure of my recovery, but Dr. Cowdrey had said they may do a bone marrow test while they had me there. This was reliant on my counts showing sufficient improvement however. The bone marrow biopsy would reveal how my body had responded to the first bout of chemotherapy. It would tell us if my cancer was still present or if it had gone into remission. The thought of even going back to hospital unsettled me, as did the prospect of another bone marrow biopsy. The procedure had been more uncomfortable than painful. Dr. Woodward had numbed the area around my hip before pushing a needle into the bone which you can imagine takes some persuasion. The worst part without question was when he then extracted the bone marrow, which was a horrible, emptying feeling quite unlike anything else. I think I described it to someone at the time as feeling like he was sucking out my soul.

I was due at the hospital at 10.30 a.m. the following day so I needed to get myself mentally prepared.

Wednesday May 21 2008. Course 1: Day 27.

I was not prepared. We were up, showered, dressed, fed, ready to go, but I was not prepared. Mary dropped me at the front door of the hospital and went off to park the car. Luckily for us, she had a staff parking permit for the hospital car parks which was probably going to save us an exorbitant amount of money in fees by the time this was all over.

I stood outside the foyer waiting for her. By now I had started getting 'the look' from people. It's the look we reserve for people who are obviously bald through chemotherapy. If you didn't realise that we, as a species, have 'a look' for this, now you know. It's very specific and betrays a number of emotions, even though it lasts little over a second. It goes like this: a person notices you, in the sense they become aware someone is there, and their eyes move up to your face. Nothing uncommon so far, we all do this hundreds of times every day. They get a sense that something is wrong and it causes their gaze to be held on you just a split second longer than it naturally would. It's in this fraction of a moment that they reveal themselves, and you can read their mind. Their first thought is something like "Oh, that's sad," which in my case that is usually coupled with "That's no age to have cancer." Then sometimes something nice happens. Some o f them give you an almost imperceptible smile. It happens in their eyes really, and I find it's more common in older people. It seems to say "Good luck". All this happens in no time at all but you can read it as clearly as you are reading these words now. I have absolutely no problem with people giving me *the look*. Mary had told me on occasions that people were staring and that it was making her angry but I didn't mind. It's a natural thing for people to do and you can't hold it against them. That's not to say I never felt self-conscious because at times I did. I would put on a hat and just want to be normal again, be just another face in the crowd. But for the most part I was comfortable with it. This was what was happening to me and it will be a cold day in hell before I would give the cancer the satisfaction of feeling ashamed about it.

I could see Mary approaching and I suddenly became aware of the parking ticket machine by the door, where people would pay the balance on their ticket before returning to their cars. It was automated with a woman's voice, which would announce the amount you owed. I began to laugh. The emphasis and intonation in the voice was all wrong, and the disembodied voice would stress a syllable at random so strongly it bordered on extreme excitement. It was so ridiculous I couldn't help but laugh. I let go of the stress and worry I was feeling. Why carry it? What will be will be. I smiled and took Mary's hand and we went inside.

I had been advised of the quickest route to Cavendish Ward by Dr. Cowdrey, before I was discharged, but I had forgotten it so we just followed the signs from the front door. We filed slowly into the Green Zone, where Cavendish Ward was to be found the signs assured us. Sure enough there it was, and busy it was too. Around 20 people were waiting in the reception area and only a couple more seats remained. We announced ourselves to reception and took the seats but a nurse appeared at once and invited us to wait in the chemotherapy suite. "It's much more comfortable in there" she beamed. She was right. It was filled with armchairs, books and magazines giving it a feel of a nursing home's common room. One wall was lined with leaflets about various cancers and I spotted one on Acute Myeloid Leukaemia looking down on me as we took our seats. In no time Alison Galloway, the sister from Durrant Ward, came to find me. She had such a kind smile and caring nature, it was impossible not to like her. She had called in to see me several times during my stay on Durrant Ward, usually with the doctors on their rounds, and I and my family had warmed to her instantly. Knowing she was seeing me today put me at ease.

Mary and I went through to a treatment room and I climbed onto the bed while answering Alison's questions about how I was feeling and how we were coping with things. She said she was going to take some blood out of my Hickman line for the sample. This was a small mercy I had not expected. While in hospital my forearms had become a mess from the regular blood lettings. They were bruised and I had hardened veins in places. The veins themselves, when regularly accessed, do not announce themselves as obviously making it harder for phlebotomists to find them, meaning they sometimes miss causing more bruising etc, etc. and it becomes something of a vicious circle. But after a few days on the outside, and with some platelets of my own doing a repair job, my arms now looked pretty much normal. Still, to be told I was being spared another needle was something. Despite this, I remembered that my doctors had passed comment on blood samples obtained through the Hickman line and how they sometimes produced a skewed result. I did not know the reason for this being so, but wanted the doctors to get an accurate reading of what was going on in my blood. But the decision had been made to use the Hickman line so Alison took the sample, before flushing the line through to keep it clean and changing the nozzles that dangled and flapped on the end, constantly reminding me I had a cable sticking out of my chest. We were advised to return in 45 minutes, when one of my doctors would go through the results. We knew the ward was very busy that day and thought that might be an ambitious timescale, but agreed to return and wait in the chemo suite. As we left the ward, we spotted Drs. Cowdrey and Strong buzzing from room to room, picking up patient files and disappearing through doors. This was the business of what they did.

We went to the canteen to silence the beast of my hunger, and leisurely make our way back to the ward. Inside the chemotherapy suite, a middle-aged man was hooked up to a drip and I deduced he had probably had a chemo drug pushed through it. We sensed we were in for a wait, so tried to compile which questions we needed to ask. We read, I ate, I stewed. It was a further hour on top of the 45 minutes we were advised before Dr. Cowdrey breezed in with an apology, but minus the smile I had seen him wearing the last few times we had met. I knew instantly something was wrong. He asked me about my health and the vagaries of my bowel movements. I gave curt replies, trying to steer him towards the results of my blood test. Essentially, Dr. Cowdrey said, my white cells were still climbing albeit not at an accelerated rate, and my platelets were also on the up. My red cells, however, which transport oxygen around the body, had dropped. This was probably due to the fact that it had now been several days since my last transfusion and all those cells were now done for. The red cells I had were my own, I just didn't have as many as I did a few days ago. I was crestfallen. It was too early to do the bone marrow test, Dr. Cowdrey said. I never thought I would be disappointed not to be having one of those. "What I'm going to recommend" Dr. Cowdrey said, "is that you come back in a week and we repeat the test." "A week!" I screamed in my head. "A week!" All I could find to say out loud was "Oh". Dr. Cowdrey was still talking "Make yourself an appointment for a week today and we'll see how we're looking then." Mary asked a question while I stared into space. It was a pertinent one: about the cytogenetic test results we had not been party to. These were tests on my chromosomes which would reveal if I was at low, standard or high risk of not responding to chemotherapy. Dr. Cowdrey said he too had not seen any results and it was something which needed to be chased up. I continued to stare into space as Dr. Cowdrey closed my file and left, leaving Mary and I in a hole where we didn't know quite what to say. I instantly thought of our wedding – so delicately placed on the time line of my treatments and recoveries that bandying around periods of time like a week could so easily throw the whole thing off. It could mean I was still too ill for the ceremony to go ahead, or make me one week weaker on the day. Perhaps Dr. Cowdrey had forgotten the time pressures we were working to. I wasn't sure I had a week.

We made our way off the ward and Alison called to me, "Are you not having a bone marrow test, Richard?" I explained what Dr. Cowdrey had told me, and Alison did her best to play it down as normal, though I sensed it was not good news. All the appointments were full for the following week, but the receptionist had no choice but to keep adding names between the lines. So many people going through the same worries we were. We made our way back towards the car in a stunned silence. Mary was trying to reassure me over what had just happened, but my head was filling with questions. My counts must have been a long way below what was expected for Dr. Cowdrey to send me away for a week. Why not just a day or two, if I was anywhere in touching distance? Why weren't my cells coming back faster? Did I still have a high presence of cancerous cells which were slowing the production of healthy cells? These are the questions you don't think of until afterwards, and they were weighing heavy on my mind.

It was as we talked, crossing the car park hand in hand, that something happened. I think it was just at the moment I decided that worrying accomplished nothing, and all I could do was concentrate on recovery, that it hit me. I felt the strength come back into my legs. It was sudden, like someone had flicked a switch, sparking failed floodlights back into life and sending the crowd into raptures. Until that moment I had been unsteady on my feet and unable to walk very far at all. Suddenly, I felt, that had changed, but I didn't want to pass comment at first in case it left me as quickly as it had returned. We walked back past the entrance of the hospital and out to the far car park, so far so good.

I told Mary I wanted to go somewhere and we drove to the town centre and parked up. Dr. Cowdrey had told me to avoid places that were very crowded, but said there was no reason I couldn't walk around town. At the time, that was beyond my imaginings. I told Mary we would just have a look in a few shops and see what I could manage. I surprised us both. Three hours later, I was still going strong.

Thursday – Saturday: May 22 – 24 2008. Course 1: Days 28 - 30.

I felt I had turned a corner. Getting my strength back was a huge piece of the psychological jigsaw of recovery. I wasn't now dancing on any tabletops, even stairs were an obstacle, but I could function much more independently. The weakness I had felt in hospital was one of the most depressing elements. Not having the energy to drag myself from my bed was immensely upsetting to me. Needless to say, it was also very limiting. How much of it was down to my counts and how much was malnutrition I couldn't say, but I had quickly put on several pounds in weight since leaving hospital. For the next couple of days we were able to do more. I could go with Mary to do jobs or pay bills, or to buy birthday cards. Life could be lived more or less normally. I had to keep telling myself to take it easy though. I may have felt stronger but my legs had been called upon to do very little in the past few weeks and they didn't always do as they were told. I would occasionally begin walking off at an unintended angle or have a wobble and have to catch my balance. I had one such scare at the very top of a department store escalator, where I had foolishly taken my hand off the rail. I suddenly lost my balance and lurched backwards, but managed to regain my composure. It was a good reminder of my limitations, even though it scared the shit out of Mary and me.

Some of our days are quite busy now I was mobile. Lots of people wanted to see us and there were lots of people we wanted to see, sometimes the lists even tallied. Mary kept a watchful eye on me and made sure I wasn't exerting myself. "We should only do what you're comfortable with" she told me. "If we have to cancel, people will understand." But I was feeling good, and wanted to do more. I had been quarantined for a month and, now I was out, everything looked, tasted, smelled and felt better than before. I would put on an old CD and be absolutely captivated by it. Was it me or did it sound even better than before? Life was more vivid and it was more precious. I wasn't about to take rest days thank you very much. Being told I had cancer, and the time I had been afforded to reflect upon that, had had a very orderly effect on my thoughts. While one might expect such a bombshell to send a mind into chaos, to launch it into frenzy; with me it had quite the opposite effect. I was as calm as could be. Zen almost, if you care for that sort of thing. News of such gravitas had ordered my thoughts and priorities, and I was left with a very clear and tidy space up top. My other cares and worries were banished, and I had a very definite sense of what was important. It is the people we love who matter; it is our health and our happiness. Everything else is a bonus. Little niggles and problems not to mention most of the big ones do not matter. We all know this on some level. I know I am saying nothing revolutionary; it's just that it is so hard to surrender that weight we carry. For me, and several of my closest family and friends, this was no longer a problem. Irritations and trivialities were lost on the wind. That was one of the blessings of all of this.

While I may have been feeling better and stronger each day, I could see that Mary was feeling the strain. Although I was calling upon her less and less to help me do things, she was not sleeping well and I sensed she was more worried about me than she was letting on. Mary is a natural worrier, but since all this began she had been so strong and positive, which had got me through no end of low times. I had been called on to reassure her a few times, but for the most part, to my face at least, she had been rock solid. Now though, she was tired and the cracks were starting to show. She would snap at me or get worked up over something small, then feel guilty and apologise. I didn't help matters because I'm stubborn and would automatically argue back rather than try to get to the root of the problem. Things were simmering for the whole day and it wasn't until late on, when we were in the car on our way home from a meal out, that Mary finally opened up. She was feeling very tired and emotionally drained. The more she got that way, the more worried she felt about me. In her mind, she had to confront the possibility that she may lose me. The success of my treatment was by no means guaranteed. She was scared, but felt she had to hold it together for me. "I just don't want you to ever leave me" she said, crying now. It was hard to know what to say in return. I could make no promises, so I just said something that I believed to be true. "What is happening to us, all this, is just an obstacle. It's not the end."

Sunday May 25 2008. Course 1: Day 31.

Although I was now enjoying deeper, more restful sleeps, some nights were still eventful. I was obviously troubled by bad dreams and waking nightmares, though I had no memory of them come morning. Mary would tell me how I would toss and turn and sweat, or sit up and point at ghosts. I would talk. I would wake Mary, when I was somewhere on the outskirts of sleep, and urge her to look at things which weren't there, becoming angry when she suggested I go to sleep. This did little to ease either Mary's tiredness or my concerns about my mental health. Mary had tried one of her Diazepam tablets for the first time, but I ranted and raved so much during that night it was anything but restful for her. I hoped this would be something that would settle down. After all it was not unheard of for me to do such things occasionally, albeit it not to the extent seen here.

We busied ourselves during the day by seeing family. Mary confessed she was getting sick of thinking about food and arranging meals to feed my insatiable appetite, which was showing no signs of abating. Our plans had to fit around mealtimes, when I would put away an awful lot of food, which was becoming expensive. We both knew it was necessary though. Soon I would be back on those chemo drugs and my appetite would be a thing of the past.

As it was a Sunday Mary asked me if I would like to go to church with her that evening for Mass. Mary and all her family, which is very large, are Catholic. I, on the other hand, come from atheist stock. This had never caused us any arguments. We respected each other's beliefs and I was happy for our wedding to include or comprise the full Catholic service. Mary had invited me to attend a Mass with her before, but I had always declined. Apart from one service I could remember from my primary school days, the only times I had attended church were for weddings or funerals. But I knew my name had been passed to the priest at the Annunciation, where we were due to marry in September, and the congregation had been asked to pray for me. The least I could do was go along.

Something about churches scares me. They always have. Whatever one's beliefs, walking into a church, has an effect on the soul. There is an atmosphere that is humbling and, for me, unsettling. Basically, I am afraid I'll melt. I'm scared that, actually, there is a God and he's none too impressed with the way I've been carrying on. It was the day before the Bank Holiday Monday which usually saw me getting completely bladdered in the hostelries of our fair town, a far cry from Sunday Mass. But the offer was there and I said I would go, for Mary's benefit. "It's to your benefit as well you know," she said. "You're the one who's sick." I said it would be somewhat hypocritical for me to start asking God for things now. Mary replied that "It doesn't work like that". We parked up outside and I began to get the fear that I might be struck down by a bolt of lightning, it had come over rather cloudy. But I made it inside unscathed and Mary collected some little booklets we would need, dipped her finger in some water and touched it to her forehead. We took our seats and the Priest began to speak. Periodically, everyone would say things in chorus and it was all a bit like the workings of a secret society. They all stood up, they all sat down. "And also with you," they said. At one point, everyone around me began shaking hands with everyone else, which was all very welcoming, if unexpected. Mary went up to receive some bread from the priest, and I was left alone on the back row with my thoughts. I looked at the statue of Jesus at the front of the church. I watched the people around me showing their devotion and receiving comfort in return. Did I believe in these peoples' God? No, I couldn't say I did, even in this, my hour of need. But I was open to faith. The idea that there is some benevolent force in the universe, binding everything together, is not something I would dismiss. Though I don't subscribe to any religion, perhaps that core value, which essentially they share, was feasible to me. Or maybe I was just reaching, because I was scared. Even if this force existed, why would it take notice of me? In recent weeks we had witnessed a cyclone in Burma and an earthquake in China. Thousands of people had died, thousands more were dying. There would be an infinite number of prayers more urgent and desperate than my own to listen to. Still, I could but try. There, on the back row of the church, while everyone else queued to receive Eucharist, I bowed my head and closed my eyes and asked for something I thought was fair. I didn't want any help getting through this. I didn't ask to be well. I asked for enough time, and I hoped that whoever I was speaking to would know what I meant.

Tuesday May 27 2008. Course 1: Day 33.

It was the day before my hospital appointment for a blood test and, potentially, another bone marrow biopsy. I lay in bed thinking about what it may reveal. The bone marrow test would say whether my cancer was in remission, which was clearly going to be a massive piece of news. I could envisage myself bursting into tears either way. I didn't feel as though

I was in remission, but what I was basing this on I couldn't say. Instinct just told me I wasn't. I considered things for a few minutes and then sat up to face another day. As I did so I was hit by a wave of sadness and doubt that pinned me to the mattress. Mary came in, right on cue. She had amazed me throughout this whole process, the way she had always appeared just when I needed her. She always knew just how much help to give, sensing when I wanted to attempt things myself and when I needed a hand but was too proud to ask. Here she was again, just when I needed her. She sat with me and I put my head on her shoulder and started to cry. I didn't need to explain why. Mary reassured me, but confessed that she too was nervous about tomorrow. If my blood test showed my cells were recovering poorly we wouldn't need a bone marrow biopsy to tell us things weren't looking good. We talked for a few minutes, but I couldn't shake the sadness off. Then Mary asked me the question I had hoped she would never ask – "What are you most afraid of?" I told the truth. "I'm frightened for you if I'm not going to be here," I said. Her eyes suddenly filled with tears. "People lose people every day" she told me. "They go out to work and they never come back. But we're going to be okay because we've been given this chance. We've been given this opportunity to make you better, and there's just no room for you thinking negatively." She was right of course, and I tell her that and I say I'm sorry. I've been so positive through all this and I'm angry at myself for slipping, as though my doubts would feed the cancer. I ask to be left alone for a minute to get myself together. When she returns, Mary looks at me and I see her deflate. She shakes her head "Richard, you look terrified" she said. We spend the rest of the day shopping for wedding rings. We end up spending more than double what we had set aside for them. Because fuck it, that's why.

Wednesday May 28 2008. Course 1: Day 34.

I wake up early and make a dash for the bathroom. For the second morning in a row I find a big puddle on the laminate floor around the toilet. Again I look to see if it has leaked, or if there are patches where it has come through the ceiling. It has not, which leaves me with one alternative; I must be urinating on the floor during the night like some untrained Alsatian. I have no memory of doing this, but it requires no leap of the imagination given my behaviour of late and the number of times I have to wander to the bathroom in a stupor during the night. Disgusted with myself, I tell Mary what I think has happened and she tells me not to worry; I am ill and under massive amounts of stress. These things happen, she tells me. As supportive as she is being, it can't be nice for her to know her fiancé has taken to marking his territory about the house like some feral tomcat. Where next after the bathroom? The bedroom? The kitchen? It's not something we needed on the morning of my hospital appointment.

We headed off in good time and I found it easy to get into the right frame of mind. I was feeling positive about the tests. Something in me just told me they were going to give us good news, that we were due some good news. We took our seats in the waiting room and expected a long wait. I soon spotted both Drs. Strong and Cowdrey working their way through the many assembled patients, and both said hello as they passed. I heard my name called at the other end of the corridor and I went off to announce myself. A nurse asked me to follow her for my blood test. When we passed where Mary was sitting, I saw she was talking with Dr. Cowdrey. "Ah Richard," he said. "I was just telling Mary that we got back the results of your cytogenetic tests." I braced myself. These were the tests on my chromosomes to determine how pre-disposed I was to responding to chemotherapy. Dr. Cowdrey went on: "The results show you are in the standard risk category, so we are straight down the middle of the road." I let go of the breath I now realised I had been holding. It was good news. As long as I wasn't in the High Risk category there was nothing which would have a bearing on my treatment or give cause for concern. I thanked Dr. Cowdrey and he marched off purposefully down the corridor. Mary and I smiled at each other. It was a relief to know the results of the cytogenetics test at long last, as they had been hovering for some time. It only added to my positive feeling about the day, and I was convinced it would not be the last piece of good news we would receive. The nurse took me into a side room and took a sample of blood from my Hickman line, before cleaning and flushing the line through.

Mary and I decided to take a walk to the canteen and leave at least an hour before returning for the test results, as the ward did seem especially busy. I was still eating an awful lot of food, and snacking right up until going to bed. Sometimes, even in bed. I had also developed a real sweet tooth, which was funny because I ate savoury food almost exclusively before all this began. I guessed it was my body trying to gain weight, and I had to admit this constant gluttony was fun. The way I saw it, I would soon be back in hospital with no appetite and no sense of taste, so it would be foolish not to feast before the famine. Mary watched me eat my mid-morning snack of a jacket potato with chilli, a chocolate brownie and chocolate bar, and then we slowly made our way back to the ward.

As it turned out, we didn't have long to wait before Dr. Cowdrey craned his neck around the corner and invited us into his office. I searched his face for the smile that always gave away if he was sitting on good news. Just as I took my seat, I spotted it flash across his face. He spoke, asking me about my health and whether the allergic rash I had developed in hospital had gone. I confirmed that it had, and gave brief answers to his other questions, keen to know what was happening in my blood. "Right," he began. "It's good news. Your blood is almost normal. Your haemoglobin levels are good, the platelet count is excellent and white cell count is borderline for us to start the second treatment." I felt like punching the air and celebrating in the manner a sozzled football fan might mark a crucial goal. But I didn't have Dr. Cowdrey down as a football fan, so I just beamed a smile in an exceedingly restrained fashion. Dr. Cowdrey went on: "The way your blood has responded is indicative of the cancer being in remission, but we won't know until we've don't a bone marrow test, which I'm proposing we do right away." Even a thought of one of those wasn't going to bring me down. I was flying. I signed the form consenting to the bone marrow, and Dr. Cowdrey left us in his office while he went to get the room ready. I looked over at Mary and took her hand. I was the happiest I had been in weeks and saw the light at the end of the tunnel grow all the brighter. Mary, although happy, was more subdued than I was, and I quickly realised the news had hit her as relief, rather than joy and excitement I was feeling. We now knew I was to be readmitted on Tuesday to begin the next course of treatment.

This gave me another six days grace on the outside but ate into our timescale for the wedding. We had worked out that, allowing a full four weeks for recovery after each chemo, I would reach something like a peak in health for September 12, our wedding day. That was assuming, however, I started the second course on the day previous to the date I had been given. Such long breaks between courses, though pleasurable, were something I could not afford if I was to be on top form on the big day.

When Dr. Cowdrey was ready I followed him into a side room with one of the nurses who was to assist. I deliberately didn't look at the apparatus tray. There was nothing to be gained from that as far as I could see. So, despite undergoing this procedure twice, I still had no idea how thick the needle was. Dr. Cowdrey told me he performed the procedure slightly differently to Dr. Woodward, who had carried out the first one. I'd be lying on my side this time, with my knees up near my chest. Dr. Cowdrey said: "I won't be taking any bone sample this time, so the procedure should be less painful, in theory." I assumed the position, lowered my waistband, and then wondered why he had added "in theory". The nurse commenced with the small talk. She was nice enough, but I knew if she persisted with it when there was a needle in my bone I would be less cordial. Dr. Cowdrey warned me he was about to inject the Lignacaine anaesthetic, using the same "sharp scratch" terminology that all the blood suckers employed. He left the needle in for a long time, spreading the anaesthetic around. The whole area was quickly numbed but the needle kept making contact with my hip bone, which was the only unpleasant part thus far. I was still locked in small talk with the nurse when Dr. Cowdrey told me to get ready for the other needle, which signalled the end of our conversation as far as I was concerned. Just as before, I felt nothing until it pressed onto my hip bone. Dr. Cowdrey pressed hard and, I think, turned the needle to burrow in. I'm not sure of this, as I was facing away, but that is what it felt like. The pressure on the bone was more unpleasant than painful, and I was now replying to the nurse's questions with winces only. "Well," Dr. Cowdrey remarked. "You have really hard bones." Great, I thought. That is beneficial in almost every situation life can throw at you. Except for a bone marrow biopsy, where it just complicates matters. You really want marsh mallow bones if you're intent on having one. Despite my apparent bone hardness, Dr. Cowdrey had reached the required depth and told me to brace for the sharp pain of him drawing out the fluid. I clenched my fists. It lasted only a second, but was as nasty as I remembered. "We're done. You did well," Dr. Cowdrey said as all my muscles relaxed into the bed. He took the time to see that I was okay, put his hand on my back and told me how well I was doing with everything. It was unexpected but really reassuring. I thanked him and he headed off with my sample which, again, I didn't much care to see. Some things I can live with not knowing. The nurse checked the dressing on my wound, which again was no bigger than a red dot administered by a felt tip pen. The bone would hurt later in the day but for now was painless. When Mary and I reached the car I told her "I am now almost normal – it's official." "Darling," she said. "You will never be normal."

We called in to see my dad and Marion to break the good news, and I managed to blag another meal. When we got home, I could hear a tapping sound as I took off my coat. Following my ears to the bathroom, I saw a steady stream of drips coming through the light fitting and leaving a big puddle on the laminate floor. We had a leaking roof and must have had for days, but there was no clue on the bathroom ceiling. Mary arrived on the scene. Such domestic emergencies would usually have sent her into hysteria, but with the day we'd had, what did it really matter? She grabbed a bucket and stuck it under the flow of drips, before putting both arms around me. "At least we know it's not you!"

Thursday – Saturday: May 29 – 31 2008. Course 1: Days 35 - 37.

I look a bit daft, I tell Mary. Some of the hairs on my head have started to grow back, while I have large areas which are still bald. I've been lucky really. Yes I lost most of the hair on my head but still have my body hair and, most importantly, my eyebrows. If and when they go, that's when you really look like a cancer patient. I asked Mary to shave my head again. Having everything at a consistent length looks better I decide. I found I was wearing a hat for most of the time I am outside or in company and I try to understand why I am doing this. I do feel slightly self-conscious about the baldness, but I think it runs deeper than that. I think I just want people to behave in a normal way towards me. Sometimes I go to pick something up and someone will try to take it off me or ask if I can manage. I don't begrudge them that – it is done with the best of intentions, I just don't want to be treated as an invalid or as though I am sick. Occasionally I'll catch someone looking at my dome head. That's fine too. I was still getting used to it myself. It just served as a reminder, to them and me, about what was going on. I had come to terms with my illness and what was ahead. I was remaining positive and buoyant for the majority of the time, but the only way I was maintaining this was by thinking about it as little as possible. My condition was never far from my thoughts or from rearing its head in conversation, but I couldn't allow it to become too absorbing. Mentally, I needed enough of a break from thinking about haemoglobin and Cytarabine. Acting normally and looking normal, helped to accomplish this.

I had contacted our insurers to try and make a claim for the hole in the roof, citing storm damage. My dad and I had been up in the loft, and spent half an hour taking it in turns to peer through the darkness with a torch. Then Mary poked her head up through the hatch, and asked why we didn't just put the light on. She pulled the cord neither of us had seen and the roof space was filled with light. It was a surprisingly large room, and Mary soon began with ideas about converting it. I didn't want to burst her bubble by asking where exactly we would factor in another staircase. My dad soon found the hole, through which rain water was coming in at a steady rate. Our house had an old fashioned slate roof, and it was clear several of the tiles had been disturbed by the wind. Daylight shone through in a few other areas but the roof seemed to be keeping out the rain in everywhere but one spot. If we had a magic wand, a whole new roof would have been preferable but this was so far beyond our finances it was hardly worth talking about. We did a bit of temporary shoring up of the roof. By this I mean we stuffed one of those tough blue bags used for recycling newspapers into the hole and waited. After a few minutes, the water coming through into the bathroom slowed. We took the light fitting off in the bathroom and the silver base was completely full of water. The weather forecast was for dry conditions for the next couple of days and we had been told we could expect the inspector from the insurance company in two days time. I just had to hope I could convince him the hole was not general wear and tear, otherwise our fund was about to have a big bite taken out of it.

Sunday June 1 2008. Course 1: Day 38.

I woke late, though still with the feeling I could have slept much longer. We had friends over the night before and sat out in our modest back yard talking about everything except any diseases any of us may have had, which suited me fine. It was the first time since my treatment that I had fancied a beer. Up until then the thought of drinking had strongly disagreed with me. I only had three, over the course of several hours, so the alcohol couldn't reasonably be blamed for my lethargy in the morning. It was more my mood weighing me down. I felt bogged down by a feeling I couldn't describe. It lay somewhere between sadness, anger and fear but wouldn't settle in any of those camps. I tried to get on with the day and busy myself in something potentially cathartic in its mundaneness, like washing up or sweeping the back yard. Mary was quiet too, and as much as she may protest, she is never quiet when all is well. We moved about the house like ghosts of each other, occasionally asking the other what was wrong. But in our efforts to put a brave face on things, we would each reply that we were fine. This bare-faced lie would of course anger the other, who was not so astute as to realise we were both going through the same ritual. As was bound to happen eventually, we were both having a down day, and we weren't there to pick the other up. One of us needed to make the first move. I had gone back to bed when Mary came to find me. She asked me to sit up and give her a hug and, as I did, I fell apart. I cried for a long time, and then started again when I thought I was finished. Despite this release, I couldn't really say what was behind it. We went out for a walk and I felt really drained. Tomorrow was to be my last 24 hours of freedom. The weather forecast predicted lots of rain. I think we were both glad when we crawled into bed and the day was over.

Monday June 2 2008. Course 1: Day 39.

We were due visits from two inspectors about our leaky roof, one checking for internal damage and one for external damage. I was also expecting a visit from my editor, who had arranged to call round in the afternoon. First to arrive was Mr. Internal who busied himself taking photos of the hole where our bathroom light fitting had once been fixed. He talked at 100 mph, telling me they would look at the electrics, and re-do the ceiling if it had been water-damaged. He punched details into a hand-held computer while I stood there staring at the hole or my feet, waiting for him to finish. He said they would be in touch and I showed him out.

Knowing it was my last day out, Mary and I had some things to do. We were making our own wedding invitations and, after settling on a design some weeks ago, had begun the first few stages. There is nothing so guaranteed to drive a wedge between couples as making them take part in craft activities, and we fell out practically every time we had even talked about them. But we had to grasp the nettle and make some, because I would soon be back in hospital and a few weeks could easily slip by unnoticed. Most of our arguments over the making of the invitations stemmed from the fact that I can be a perfectionist when it comes to such things, and I insisted on doing or overseeing everything. This was despite having cocked-up myself by cutting a load of card to the wrong size.

It was a beautiful sunny day so we sat outside and began our production line. I thought nothing of it when my dad phoned, we had been in contact every day since I was taken ill, but the tone in his voice was different. "I've just had a call from Dr. Cowdrey" he said. A thousand crises theories flashed behind my eyes. Had my test results showed something abnormal? Did I need to come back in now? My dad went on somewhat reluctantly, not wanting to be the one who broke the news. "He says there is a diarrhoea bug on Durrant Ward so it's not safe to get you in. The ward is closed to try to contain the infection." My heart was in my shoes. If there was an ongoing diarrhoea bug the problems would be two-fold. 1: if I caught it, I would be glued to the toilet all day and the chemo drugs would pass through me and not have their full effect. 2: in the fullness of time, as my immune system was destroyed by the chemo, I would be wide open to the infection and it could be potentially much more serious. But I had a more pressing problem. We had calculated the timescale of treatment and rest periods up until the wedding, and then re-done it when my first spell of convalescence dragged on. It showed the wedding day, September 12, was still in reach. Just. I could be clear of chemo and reasonably recovered, though there was hardly a day to spare. We needed things to run smoothly to have a chance of making the date. I looked down at the half-made wedding invitations carrying the date September 12 and sighed at the irony of the phone call's timing. It felt like our wedding had just been derailed.

Tuesday June 3 2008. Course 1: Day 40.

We had already discussed alternative dates with our wedding reception venue and other parties like the photographer and chauffer company, but even having dialogue about it made me feel sick. Even imagining that we may have to rearrange the wedding literally turned my stomach. It was important to us both that I was well on the day, but changing the date, to me, felt like conceding something. I felt like the cancer would already have swallowed six months of my life by the time it was over, not to mention what it may cost me later down the line health-wise. That was our wedding date and I would not relinquish it without a scrap. The problem was that there was no way of knowing for how long Durrant Ward would be closed. Every extra day spent combating the infection was eating into our chances of making the date. As far as I knew, it could be closed for a week or more.

Dr. Cowdrey had told me to come in to see him in clinic the following day, where we could discuss the situation further and I could have my Hickman line flushed. We intended to take in our calendar and ask whether we were being too ambitious. If he told me I couldn't now recover in time then I would have to find a way to accept it. But I would not rearrange just because he said it would be a stretch. I would make it. I would stretch. The delay in getting me back in had broadsided us both. We were both so disappointed, but I tried to remain upbeat for Mary's sake. She was very much of the mould of a girl who had dreamed of a perfect wedding day, the best day of her life. I was not going to be the person to say our plans may be sunk, even though I feared they were headed for an iceberg.

There was little else we could do other than enjoy what time we had together on the outside, while hoping, conversely, that it didn't last too long. We headed out in the car to pick up Mary's wedding ring from the jewellers and have a look round the shops to kill some time.

Mary had been doing all the driving whenever we went anywhere, mainly because I didn't know if I was supposed to be behind the wheel. My doctors hadn't told me I couldn't drive but there were lots of things they hadn't warned me off which I probably shouldn't do.

By now I was feeling pretty much in total health. My legs had their strength back and I could manage to do everything I would normally, except perhaps going for a run. I felt a little guilty for being off work, in what had developed into a little holiday at the end of my first treatment. That coming Sunday I would have been out of hospital for three weeks. But I resolved to never punish myself for feeling good, nor take it for granted. The days of being unwell were still very clear in my memory and I knew that many more were to come. Each and every day that I was able, from that until my last, had to be grasped and made to matter. We had just picked up Mary's ring when my dad called me on my mobile. He told me he had just spoken to the haematology sister, Alison Galloway, who had said that, as far as she was concerned, it was safe for me to come in the following day. I was to wait for a phone call in the morning telling me when to make my way in. It was the news we had been hoping for. If I could get started again tomorrow then the wedding date may still be within reach. My dad went on: "The ward is being steam cleaned and is being inspected in the morning, so it may be the afternoon before you get in."

Back at home I began packing my things while Mary called Durrant Ward to request they call my mobile rather than my dad's number, meaning he didn't have to wait by the phone. She spoke to one of the nurses we had become friendly with, who, not knowing how much we had been told let slip that the diarrhoea bug was, in fact, C-diff. That explained the precautionary measures. The infection, the same that had closed neighbouring Eastwood Ward, is particularly nasty and potentially deadly. The nurse told us that the plan was to keep the ward closed other than for myself and a man aged 30, who had been diagnosed over the weekend. The ward would be manned by one member of staff. Mary told me that, from the way the nurse was talking, they thought it unlikely they would be cleared by Infection Control by tomorrow. These revelations put a new spin on things. How desperate was I to get back into hospital, enough to run the gauntlet with C-diff? I also began to think of this 30 year old man, going through the dark uncertainty of these first days against a backdrop of a superbug outbreak. I wanted to talk to him. I wanted to give him the benefit of my limited experience or answer any of his questions if I could. I wanted to tell him everything would be okay, as futile as it would probably sound. But I knew that with the necessary containment procedures for both of us we would probably never meet though we would spend months just doors apart. Mary, too, had been affected by hearing of the man's admission, and had been transported back, vividly, to a terrifying point in our time-line. Some old feelings, not yet dealt with, resurfaced and for the rest of the night she was upset and had a far-off look in her eye.

Wednesday June 4 2008. Course 1: Day 41.

I had become rather good at waiting. Spending a month in hospital guarantees that one becomes accomplished in hurrying along spare hours. Mary, however, does not wait well. She paced and pouted as I serenely rechecked my bags. Where was the phone call? Morning had slid into afternoon and we had had no word of when it would be safe for me to come in. "I'm going to call them," Mary said. I shook my head and smiled. "They will ring us soon. Let them do what they need to do." We argued the point for another couple of minutes. I lost. The phone rang for some time before someone picked it up. Mary had that tone in her voice. "Hello, its Richard Woolley's fiancée calling." I could overhear a muffled greeting from Gavin down the receiver and pleasantries were exchanged before my better half got down to business. "We were told someone would call us in the morning to let us know what was happening but we've not heard anything." I could make out Gavin apologising, followed by a minute or so of talking, I only caught snatches of. Then I heard a sentence ring out: "We're hoping we can get him in on Friday." I closed my eyes and the sun went in. A shiver went through to my fingertips. I had heard enough. Mary extended a hand to me but I backed out of the room. What chance did our wedding have now? I had no faith in being in hospital by Friday even, the way the week had gone so far. I didn't blame anyone. I wasn't angry. This was just one of those things that happens, to show you that it wasn't such plain sailing after all. But why did it have to happen now? I had never yet questioned my leukaemia or asked "Why me?" That was irrelevant, a pointless exercise in self pity I would not entertain. To ask that question is to assume there is some fate or karma at work. There isn't. Not to my mind anyway. Cancer doesn't discriminate. It stalks nuns and murderers alike. If it gets you it's a steaming dog turd of bad luck, nothing more. Luck, good and bad, I do believe in. It's fickle and it's cruel, but it's not without a sense of humour either. This new delay was a slice of bad luck and I found myself asking how much more could be sent my way before I should put in a written complaint. I tensed every muscle in my body, as though stifling a scream, then relaxed. I breathed deeply. I could do nothing. It was what it was.

My eyes fell on a copy of one of our newspapers, which my editor had brought round for me to look at. I sunk into the sofa and opened it, absent-mindedly flicking through the pages. Mary suddenly put her head around the door and handed me my mobile. "Dr. Woodward is on the phone for you," she said. Her face didn't give much away. I stood and took the phone. "Hello, its Richard." "Hi, Dr. Woodward here," he muttered, in his typically nervous style. "Listen, I'm sorry about all this messing about with getting you in. I take it you know there has been a diarrhoea bug outbreak and we don't want to expose you to it." "I understand,"I offered back, wondering if the purpose of the call was just to apologise, something I didn't feel was necessary. "Anyway Mary was asking if we had the results of your bone marrow biopsy yet and we do." I paused. "Great," I said. "Okay what does it say?" I was rooted to the spot, but settled onto the arm of the sofa. This result would tell how well I had responded to the first course of chemo i.e. what concentration of the cancerous cells were still in my bone marrow. The magic word here was 'remission', which would mean the cancer had taken a beating and there was little or none of it to be seen under the microscope. I heard paper shuffling. "Now I know we have the result, but I don't know what it is, so you'll have to forgive me while I dig it out." I exhaled and tried to steel myself against more bad news. Mary stood, arms folded, waiting, her face etched with hope. "We haven't had the result from Sheffield yet,"Dr. Woodward said. "We send them a sample as well just as a second pair of eyes. But we do have our report back which is, er, hold on..." more shuffling. The cars on the road outside went quiet. The world stopped spinning just for a moment, and was still. "....Yes, okay. The result is remission." I repeated it, trying it on for size. "The result is remission." The world turned.

Mary clenched both fists. "That's what you wanted to hear isn't it?" Dr. Woodward asked through a laugh. I realised I had not reacted, and felt very little different. "Yes of course," I managed. "Thank you." I looked at Mary again and let out a big sigh, suddenly feeling very tired. "Just one more thing," Dr. Woodward said in true Columbo style, "I just wanted to ask you if you would like us to make enquiries into getting you into hospital in Sheffield. They've told us they don't have a bed right now but we could pursue it as an option if you wanted us to." I tried to wrench my thoughts back to the moment "Erm, well as you know, time is an issue for me" I said. "So, I suppose, yes, if there's going to be a significant wait to get in at Chesterfield". "Okay, right, fine. We'll be in touch soon then." I hung up the phone and Mary jumped on me, "How does it feel?" she asked excitedly. I took a little inward glance. "I don't know. I just feel really tired. Relief, I suppose." I felt the need to add: "I'm sorry." "Don't be sorry," she fired back. "Why are you sorry? It's brilliant news." "Because I don't feel ... how you feel now. I want to feel how you feel." "Look," she 'said, "This whole experience has been so stressful and emotional for you. This result is like a weight off you. It's okay to feel like that. Now get ready, we'll call round and tell your dad and Marion. I'm going to phone my mum." She kissed me again and bounced out of the room and up the stairs.

I dropped to the sofa and rubbed my eyes. What was wrong with me? This was the good news that made the delays seems trivial. Why was I so numb? I looked down to the open newspaper by my side and saw a photograph of a local 15 year old girl we had done an article upon recently. She had cancer, but was helping to organise a sponsored walk to raise money for research into the disease. What the article did not disclose, but I knew from talking to the reporter who wrote our story, was that her cancer had spread everywhere. To her organs, bones, limbs, everywhere, leaving her bed-bound, and in pain for most of the day. With the disease spread like that she had no chance, I knew. Whether she fully understood this or whether it had been explained to her, I couldn't say. Her cancer would not remit. It would multiply and choke her until she was dead. Where was the fairness in that? Why her and not me? I felt tears running down my face and was hit by a terrible guilt at hearing the word this girl and her parents would never hear.

Friday June 6 2008. Course 1: Day 43.

As good news as the remission result was, I was not home and dry by any stretch. I still had cancer. I still had another three courses of chemotherapy ahead. The fact that the treatment involved four courses of chemo, whether I was in remission after one or not, showed the disease could not be so easily chased away. There must have been instances, I reasoned, in which the bad cells were still present after three courses in a patient who was in remission after course 1. But to be told the cancer was in remission was all I could hope for at this stage.

Again we had packed our things, me ready for admission and Mary to stay at her parents' house while I was in hospital. We waited, neither of us particularly hopeful that today would be the day. Just after 12.00, the call came. Only it wasn't the one we were expecting. "Hello, this is Dr. Ng, a Registrar at Hallamshire Hospital in Sheffield," a woman's voice said. "We have been trying to find a bed for you at the request of your hospital and I can tell you we now have one." My stomach churned. This was very much Plan B. "We would like you to come in this afternoon, but we won't be in a position to start treatment until Monday." I sat down on the bed and rubbed my eyes. "Are you there?" Another two days down the pan, then. "Yes, I'm here," I said. Perhaps Chesterfield would be ready to take me back by Monday, but they could offer me no guarantees. The trip to Sheffield would take Mary at least 30 minutes in the car every day; double that if traffic was stacked up. The staff wouldn't know her and might restrict us to normal visiting hours, while Chesterfield had kindly turned a blind eye to people coming and going outside them. I might even be on a ward. I thought all these things, then realised I had no choice. "Okay, thank you," I said. "I will come in this afternoon." Dr. Ng explained that I had to attend that day to get my name into their computer system so that my chemo drugs would be prescribed in time for a Monday morning start. I would also need to stay in over the weekend, solely to bag my bed. That seemed pretty pointless to me, but no better options were presenting themselves at present. Mary didn't take the news well. Knowing the team, surroundings and the way things worked at Chesterfield made us feel better prepared to tackle the next course of treatment. Now those benefits had been pulled out from under us and it was like starting again.

It was only now that I had been summoned that it became real to Mary that I was going away again. We had made the most of my time at home and grown closer than ever. The thought of being separated again, being limited to sterile visits of a couple of hours was hard to take. Mary thought we may be able to negotiate my release from the Hallamshire for the weekend but I wasn't convinced. The doctor was quite insistent on the phone that I had to stay in to keep my bed. I didn't fancy two days in hospital just for fun.

I had a call from Alison Galloway, the sister on Durrant Ward. I hoped it would be to offer me a place at Chesterfield instead, but she was only warning me that the Hallamshire was going to call. She apologised for the situation. I was keen to know when I would be able to come back over. Basically, if I begin a treatment at Sheffield I would have to complete it there, meaning I would be at Sheffield for the eight days of the chemotherapy, 10 if you included the initial weekend. Then it was Alison's hope, and mine, that I could be transferred back to Chesterfield to recover.

When I started my first course of chemo, my blood cell counts were rock bottom so it was only a matter of days before I began feeling really unwell. This time round I would be starting with much healthier blood meaning it would take longer for my good cells to bottom out. After the eight days of chemo drugs I should still be well enough, and have enough of an immune system, to make the journey.

We loaded my stuff in the car and quietly made our way down the by-pass and into the city. Traffic was heavy and we arrived at the Hallamshire, an ugly and imposing tower block, just before 3 p.m. We went up to the main entrance without my things, still hopeful I may be allowed home again. Mary asked me which ward we were reporting to, at which point I realised I had forgotten to bring the piece of paper I had scribbled it on. I scratched my head. I thought I remembered being told G2 but the more I considered it the more unlikely it sounded. We looked on the board as we made our way up in the lift and saw that G floor was in fact given over to Gynaecology. Though it sounded unlikely that I had remembered correctly, I had a look round the corner at the Gynaecology ward anyway, something I'm pretty sure you can be arrested for. But, miracle of miracles, there was a sign saying that G2 was a temporary haematology ward.

The desk clerk was initially clueless when I said who I was, but a nurse who had been expecting me showed me to my bed, which was, as I had expected, in one of the bays. There was no need to isolate me until my white cells had crashed, so it would have been a luxury to have my own room. I wasn't being a snob, the reason I was apprehensive was that, on the ward in Chesterfield, a handful of patients thought night time was the ideal opportunity for shouting, screaming, singing and continual buzzer-pushing. If you don't sleep, chemotherapy very quickly becomes very hard. This I know. I could see Mary's face drop when I was shown to the ward bed, but I was determined to make the best of it. I may even prefer having the company, I thought, as I had gone a little stir crazy in my side room at Chesterfield.

In the bay were four beds leading up to a huge window with a majestic view over Sheffield. From my bed in the far corner I could see the city evolving from its past of looming brown factories and grey tower blocks, into a vibrant place once more. I had always loved the place. From above it looked just as welcoming, and surprisingly green. I was sharing the bay with two elderly chaps and a middle-aged bloke. The latter clearly had cancer, not just from his bald head but for the same sunken face and exhausted look I recognised from my bathroom mirror a month ago. He was engaged with a visitor, but soon called to me when I sat down on the bed and removed my hat, revealing we had the same barber. "Ay up lad," he said, "what's up with you?" "I've got leukaemia," I told him. "So have I. That's what I've got," he nodded solemnly. There was a silence. I didn't really know where to take the conversation next. It wasn't like I could ask "How are you finding it?" The man was still nodding. I could tell already he was Sheffield through and through. "How are you finding it?" he asked. I laughed a little involuntarily. He didn't smile. "Well there are good days and bad days." "Not for me," he said. "I've only had bad days. Everything that could go wrong has." I frowned, "Not everything. Something else can always go wrong." "They've taken some of my teeth out," he butted in, "I've had to have my Hickman line taken out because it got infected, my legs have swollen up, I've got a rash. Oh, it's terrible." I quickly took stock of what he'd just said. To have the Hickman line out and to have it refitted was a shocking prospect. He really did look like he was having an awful time with it, but his state of mind troubled me. He seemed to have a very negative outlook on everything, and that was something I hadn't been exposed to in a while. I tried to stay as upbeat as I could and surrounded myself with people who did the same. I had never even considered that I might not get better. "You'll beat it though," my neighbour added. "You're young. You'll beat it." He had stressed every 'you', implying he didn't give himself the same chances. "You will too," I replied, a bit robotically. He went back talking to his visitor and I felt a little deflated. There was no room for negativity in my head. I didn't even want to be around it.

Before I had time to ponder it too deeply, the ward sister appeared and we got chatting about what was to happen. I raised the question of the weekend, pointing out that it was something of a waste of everyone's time me being there. To my delight, she agreed, and said she would talk to the doctors about getting me out of there for a couple of days. That lifted Mary and my spirits, but we still had to get the okay from the doctors. While we waited for them to come around, a nurse came in to clean my Hickman line. She was very firm in pressing on the wound and then, afterwards remarked that it looked red. Dr. Ng appeared, an Asian woman of about 30, who had a look as well and agreed. "Hmm. Yes it does look red." I didn't like where this was going, and pointed out that I thought the redness was from being pressured. And, no, it didn't normally look like that. They weren't going to take my bloody Hickman line out. Dr. Ng had another look. In the end, I convinced them and was packed off for another two days' grace.

Course 2

Monday June 9 2008. Course 2: Day 1: Chemo Day 1.

I had spent my first night back in hospital and was already getting to know the neighbours. Across from me was Henry, or Sleepy, as my brain had nicknamed him. He would nap constantly through the day, turn in for the night about 9 p.m. and that would be it until morning. In rare moments of consciousness, Henry would burp loudly, be rude to nurses and his own visitors or turn round in surgical gown showing his bare arse to everyone. Henry was 89, and I got the feeling he wasn't too bothered what folk thought of him. I didn't know what was wrong with him medically, but there was talk of getting him off home.

To my left was 88 year old William, or Doc. He wore his glasses on the end of his nose and his catheter bag on the floor. He would read the Sheffield Star from cover to cover every day, he would watch TV wearing his headphones but otherwise keep himself to himself.

The same could not be said for Simon, my fellow-leukaemia sufferer, who looked much older than his 49 years. In fact Mary had estimated his age, rather rashly perhaps, at 70. Simon liked to complain and to moan. In the morning he was brought his medications and made the nurse wait while he counted every tablet. "Sixteen," he boomed at her. "Sixteen pills. I'll need a whole jug of water just to chuffing swallow 'em all!" Every time he had an I.V. drip or had to have blood taken he would sound off. If he couldn't sleep at night he would sit up and say: "Bloody hell. I can't chuffing get to sleep," so loud it would wake up everyone who had. Simon was nicknamed Grumpy, and probably not only by me. Grumpy would not eat hospital food, other than porridge and rice pudding, which he ate daily. He would not sleep under the sheets then complained he was cold all the time. He had moaned about the temperature so much he was eventually moved so that his bed was next to the air conditioner, which blew cold air all day. Neither he nor anyone else seemed to see a problem with this, so I kept my mouth shut. It would have been easy to see Simon as a clown, and indeed it would have helped me to distance myself from his negativity if I had. But here was a man battling the same disease as I was and evidently finding it even harder than I was. After one of Simon's rants, William said to him: "If there's one thing I've learnt in here it's that if you're strong in the head, there's a chance, you've a chance, no matter what they tell you." "I'm trying," Simon said. "When I first came in here I was rate positive, but they knock it out of you. I was rate positive but I keep losing it."

My chemotherapy prescription was delayed, and my first dose didn't arrive until the afternoon. As it was rigged up to a drip, I gazed at the liquid in the bags that would decide if I lived or died. Suddenly, starting treatment again seemed very real. It was Day 1 of the treatment so I was prescribed Daunoribicin, the red one, that I disliked most as I was always more sick on the days it was prescribed, as well as my twice-daily Cytarabine. As the chemicals slid down the

47

tube into my main vein, though I felt protective of my new-found health, I tried to recognise the truth: this treatment could take me where I wanted to go, it's just we had to go through hell to get there.

Tuesday June 10 2008. Course 2: Day 2: Chemo Day 2.

Two days in and I was already feeling sick. The creeping nausea that had wrecked my appetite during the first course was coming back. I was eating what I could, but still found it hard to get much down without retching, at least the food itself was on my side, apart from soggy toast in the mornings the hospital cuisine was miles better than what Chesterfield had to offer. I was on a couple of anti-sickness drugs and was determined not to vomit if I could possibly help it, doing so would undo some of the work done by my chemo and medications. Other than the sickness I was still mobile and well enough to be up and about and escape from the hospital for an hour out with Mary on the sly. I felt very focussed. I wanted to get through the days and do my time, concentrating on getting enough sleep and enough to eat. Both my eyes were fixed firmly on the wedding, and I thought of it often when I needed a lift.

I had never been around someone with cancer, never really seen it up close in someone I knew. My only real exposure to it came through doing stories on people with the disease. I had always rejected the use of two words when doing such stories. The first was ⊠battle', because it was a cliché and because I never really thought it accurately described what a person was going through. Now it seemed the perfect word. The best piece of advice I ever heard about writing was from an editor who gave a talk on my journalism course. He told us: "For every word there is the right moment, for every moment the right word. Write with a scalpel, not an axe." For me, 'battle' was never the right word until now. The second word I didn't use was because so many sufferers I had spoken to said they objected to it. The word, beloved of the tabloids is 'brave'. People with cancer told me, almost uniformly, they were not being brave. They were terrified but carried on and did their treatment. What else could they do? Several of my friends and family had used the word to describe me on occasion and I'd always picked them up on it. I was afraid sure enough. The treatment scared me, getting ill scared me, the demons in my head from course 1 scared me; cancer ruining my wedding scared me. But as I searched deeper I found I wasn't scared of losing. I had not once considered I wouldn't beat it. I never thought I might die. Whatever my odds, I would make it out of the fire, one of those who got away. That much I knew. Somehow.

Wednesday June 11 2008. Course 2: Day 3: Chemo Day 3.

Simon was happy. Mr. Grumpy-guts was beaming. His latest round of blood tests showed his counts were on the up again after his first course of chemotherapy. I eagerly listened in while the doctor told him his platelets, red and white cells had all surged since yesterday, much faster, I noted, than mine had returned. Why, I wondered, was a middle-aged man's system recovering more effectively than mine had? I had a few theories, maybe he had achieved a better remission than me or perhaps he started from a position of better health than I had. Whatever the reason, it just reinforced my disappointment in not bouncing back quicker, when youth was on my side.

Simon, with all the respect in the world, had as much time as he wanted to get better. I did not. I was on a time scale. But perhaps I was being too ambitious, thinking I could beat the disease in some express way. I didn't have Diet Leukaemia. Perhaps it's just the way people think today, they want to get things done quickly and easily, in a sanitised way. After all, we are all busy people and that's what we're used to. But I wasn't going to get better in my lunch hour, maybe it was time I started accepting that.

I could hear the doctors telling Simon he could probably go home the following day for a period of 10 days. Then he would be asked to begin course 2. Again, that worried me. The doctors here wanted course 2 to begin after just 10 days of rest, while I had spent more than three weeks at home. Had this hiatus allowed what remained of the cancer to re-establish itself? Later on, after he had told his family, Simon set me thinking further when he asked which kind of leukaemia I had specifically. Acute Myeloid Leukaemia breaks down into several strands or variations, each carrying its own level of risk. I realised I did not know which kind I had, though I remember asking the question more than once. I tried to recall if my doctors had side-stepped my query, and if they had, why? Did I have AML's short straw and not even know it? Simon informed me he had "the best kind of leukaemia you can get," adopting the demeanour of someone unveiling some top of the range gadget. I said I didn't know what type I had, feeling pretty stupid all of a sudden. "Oh," Simon said, bemused. "You want to ask more questions."

Thursday June 12 2008. Course 2: Day 4: Chemo Day 4.

I had felt quite troubled through the night and it marked my first vomiting episode. I had thus far managed to keep my food down through will power and a variety of anti-sickness drugs, and I foolishly hoped I might be able to continue that way. But as I lay in bed my stomach turned clean over and I just had time to grab the bowl before being violently sick several times. The feeling of sickness was pretty much constant through the day and became very tiring.

But when I woke in the morning I felt much better and had some periods where I didn't feel sick at all, though I still couldn't eat normally. Mary had really been putting in the hours, driving to Sheffield every day to see me in the afternoons and then hanging around in town until evening visiting hours. I felt guilty because it was tiring her out, but it was what she wanted. Having her there, even if we sit in silence, made us both feel whole again for a while.

By this time Mary had been signed off work for another four weeks. We had discussed her going back to work and shifts she could work around seeing me. Her pay packet normally was made up of subsidies for working unsociable hours or overtime, but with her being off sick, she was paid only the basic rate, leaving us a couple of hundred quid down each month. But we both agreed that, until the second course was done at least, we should stay as we were. When Mary came in she got the bad news out of the way. The insurance company inspectors had made their reports. Essentially, they did not buy our storm damage story. Apparently there was evidence of damp and rotting in the roof which had caused the tiles to move. We were covered for any damage inside the property under Accidental Damage, but only after we could prove we had met the cost of sorting the structural problems. No-one was living at our house at that moment and the weather had been glorious sunshine for the past week so we had given our roof little thought, given all the other stuff that was going on. "I'm sorry," Mary said. "I don't know what to say." I let out a long sigh, deflating like a wounded balloon. "How about 'Oh bollocks'," I suggested. It was no less than I was expecting, as cynical as I am about insurance companies. I would have been amazed; frankly, if there hadn't been a problem with our roof. The rest of the house was falling apart so why not that? It didn't sound a cheap job. We didn't know any roofers. Mary's dad, who can turn his hand to anything, said he would have a look and maybe see if he knew anyone. My dad thought we should just get a new roof altogether, which would have made my bank manager laugh. It was suggested we could even use some or all of the money from the F.A. Cup Final fund raiser, but Mary and I felt that went against the spirit of the event.

We took a spin out in the car to take our minds off it, stopping off for a coffee. When we got back to the ward, Henry had been sent home and Simon was readying his things to leave as well. I envied him that. When he had his prescriptions together he was wheeled past me and we exchanged messages of good luck. If, as I hoped, I got to recover in the Royal at Chesterfield from next week, we wouldn't meet again. I wouldn't know if he made it, he would become just another bald head in the faceless mass of the afflicted.

Friday June 13 2008. Course 2: Day 5: Chemo Day 5.

From being rather static, suddenly the ward was turning over lots of admissions and discharges. As I moved up the hall to the toilets, I was conscious of several empty beds but they soon began filling up again. I was over-hearing a lot of staff conversations and picked up snippets of information about various patients. I knew, for example, that the lad in Bay 2, with his left arm in plaster, had taken out his mum's car and crashed it. He looked about 15. I knew there was another man in his 50s on the ward who was just beginning the AML trial course of treatment. I knew that George, the new face in our bay, was dying. George was retirement age and had multiple myeloma. He was normally cared for at home by his wife, who was clearly devoted to him, but lately his pain had been so severe he had to be admitted to hospital. George's wife, Jane, who always dressed very glamorously, used to be a nurse and told Mary she had promised her husband he wouldn't have to see the inside of a hospital room again. George was on some heavy duty painkillers and slept for most of the time. On his first day, however, he spent a full hour staring at the ceiling, perhaps trying to spy heaven through the white tiles. It was one of the saddest things I'd ever seen and I silently begged him to go back to sleep.

Lots of visitors would come and go along the ward and couldn't resist peering in through the windows at us, the curious spectacles within. It did feel like a zoo on occasion and, just like zoo animals, sometimes we didn't want to be looked at. I remembered a visit Mary and I had made to Twycross Zoo when I had been well. A huge orang-utan had spent the whole day with a beach towel over his head. I could identify with that.

I could sense that William, in the bed alongside me, was also becoming frayed with hospital life. William was having memory lapses. I would hear him telling nursing staff he couldn't remember getting changed or moving out of bed to the chair. He couldn't remember large parts of the previous day and it was worrying him what he had been doing during these times. He asked Alec, one of the nurses, if he had been shouting or swearing, as he had done this once before at home, he confided. Alec confirmed that William, a true old-school gentleman in every sense, had been doing nothing of the sort. But William worried over this lost time, were staff keeping notes on outbursts, thinking him crazy, and not telling him? Was he crazy? Just by keeping my eyes and ears open I was exposed to a rich and ever-changing soap opera of these people's lives. *Casualty* had nothing on this place.

Saturday June 14 2008. Course 2: Day 6: Chemo Day 6.

Alison, the ward sister at Chesterfield, had told me earlier in the week that they would try and save me a bed for Tuesday. This couldn't be guaranteed of course, but we were both hopeful I could get back over there. I felt more at ease with my doctors and wanted the freedoms being in that side room afforded me with visitors. I had then raised the point with Dr. Ng when she made her rounds. I tried to phrase it in such a way so she would not be offended by my wanting to skulk off straight after the treatment. I needn't have worried. After all, we're living in the age of patient choice. She said that it should be okay, if that's what I wanted, and she would liaise with Chesterfield to see if it was possible. They wouldn't be able to give an indication until Monday, however, things moving as they do. The move was also dependant on my health. If my counts were too low, I was going nowhere. I asked Dr. Ng for some up to date news on what my blood was doing. My counts were slowly coming down, but not so fast, I thought, that it may threaten the move. But things can change, I knew. Dr. Ng then asked if I had discussed stem cell harvesting with my doctors at Chesterfield. I swallowed and stared back. As I understood it, that was last resort territory. I had not discussed it, I said. "We will give you a leaflet on what is involved. Basically, we would look to take stem cells as a precaution. There is nothing to indicate you would need them at this stage." Those were the magic words. I was all for precautions. I had to play the game. Then she went and ruined it by telling me they did it between the third and fourth courses of chemo. If it would delay the fourth course at all then it was a no-no. Didn't these people understand? I had no time for it.

Not for the first time, I wondered if my bloody-mindedness over the wedding was actually putting my life at risk. I sighed and nodded, realising I didn't have to make any decisions now. The theory was the stem cells, which had the potential to become any type of cell, would be harvested while my counts were reasonable, and not after four courses of chemo when they would likely be more sluggish. The procedure itself was rather intricate. I would be given growth injections daily for four days. This would kick-start an over-production of stem cells by convincing my body that I had flu. On the following day I would be hooked up to a machine, through which my blood would pass over the course of four hours, and stem cells would be skimmed off. I would have a needle in one arm for blood going out, and a needle in the other for blood coming back in. The use of the word 'needle' and the fact that my arms would be anaesthetised made me think they wouldn't be tickling sticks. The leaflet wasn't too comforting either. "If a suitable vein in your arm cannot be located," it said, authoritarianly "one would be found in your groin or neck." I closed the leaflet.

It was about then that I felt an uncomfortable rumble in my stomach and I quickly made for the toilet. It was as I had feared, diarrhoea. Having the squits is never just the squits when you are in hospital. Staff are always asking you: "Any diarrhoea?" with a cheery disposition. Their mood would soon change if you had. "Ooh. Right," they'd say. What follows is urine tests, stool samples, stomach examinations, etc. etc. and, at worst, lock down. Isolation. I saw their side of it, any viral element had to be contained or you ended up with outbreaks like the one at the Royal. But the isolation I had originally wanted at Sheffield now scared me. If I was put in isolation with a diarrhoea bug there is no way I could transfer to Chesterfield, no way they would accept me. I could sit there a couple of days for it to clear by which time my counts could have crashed. But I couldn't just keep the facts to myself, could I? Other people's health could be at stake, not to mention my own. I bit the bullet, owned up to the next nurse who asked. "Ooh. Right," she said. I was asked to give a urine sample and to let her know if it happened again. I grumpily shuffled back to my bed. "It's probably just a stomach upset from all the chemo drugs," Mary said confidently, "you'll be fine, don't fret over it." I huffed. "It's probably C-diff," I joked. "Imagine the irony." Mary gave me one of those wrist-slapping looks. "Richard, do not be so stupid. If you had that you would know about it. Believe me."

Sunday June 15 2008. Course 2: Day 7: Chemo Day 7.

It was Father's Day, and my dad and sister had arranged to visit me. I said we should go out somewhere rather than just crowd around my bed gawping at me like I might do a trick. My dad had agreed to this but kept saying beforehand, "Don't try and do more than you can." He, just like all my visitors, expected so little of me. I mean that in the nicest possible way, well or not, they took me as they found me. During course 1 I was more often ill than not and even had to ask visitors to leave on several occasions, or rather Mary did, always spotting when I was going downhill. The truth was that, so far, I felt more or less okay other than the feeling of sickness and an occasional stomach ache. I knew my counts were slowly coming down and were currently just below normal. Occasionally I would feel a little light-headed as a result but for the most part I was smiling and mobile. That was a big change on this time during course 1 when, having started with rock-bottom counts I was feeling like a squashed turd. That was normal, the doctors told me. Course 1 was usually the hardest, the worst. Now I was on day 7 of the 8-day second course and I had my eyes fixed on the finish line like a sprinter. Tunnel vision. This was no sprint race, though, more's the pity. Once the drugs were finished, I could look forward to a steady decline in my bloods and all the associated joys that went with it. It still took some getting used to that the drugs should take so long to work.

My recovery would be at Chesterfield if all went to plan but I wondered why I was so keen to get back there. Yes, I was happier with my doctors and Alison, but the place didn't hold many happy memories. When I walked into that room I didn't know how I would feel. Would I feel a strange affection for the place, or would it reawaken my paranoia and fear? The truth was Mary was spending a fortune on petrol and parking to visit me in Sheffield and the travelling was tiring her out. Other visitors couldn't make it over at all. That was the main reason for going back, though I did want to be off the ward by the time my immune system croaked.

I thought things over during the morning and had my chemo, Cytarabine, as usual at 10 a.m., before getting ready. Mary met me at the lifts on our way down to the lobby. The lifts at the Hallamshire are an infuriating puzzle, four metal boxes, always full, that seem to be going everywhere except where you are. Some would routinely by-pass your floor in an act of mischievousness. Just getting in them was trial enough. After pressing the 'call' button I once waited 16 minutes before setting foot in one. 10 minute waits were not uncommon. Other times the door would open and be so crammed full of people and wheelchairs, I was put in mind of an episode of *Record Breakers* I once saw involving a disabled football team and a mini. A lot of the time, we took the stairs. We met my dad at the front and jumped in Emma and her boyfriend's Dave's car and went to a cafe. I was feeling pretty good and was thankful for it. There was nothing worse than telling visitors they could come and then seeing the disappointment and awkwardness on their faces if I was out of it or quiet. We had a sit down and a catch-up for a couple of hours, which for us consisted of a good piss-taking session, one of my favourite pastimes. It was a good afternoon. It was nice to forget sometimes.

Back at the ward I had that rumble in my guts again a couple of times in the afternoon and evening and hurried down the hall to the bathroom. While the result wasn't normal, it was, I thought, some way short of diarrhoea. That afternoon I made the decision to keep my mouth shut about it, so long as it didn't get worse. It wasn't keeping me glued to the bog all day and I didn't have a temperature so it couldn't be anything viral or nasty, I thought. I was only here another day and intended on keeping my head down.

Monday June 16 2008. Course 2: Day 8: Chemo Day 8.

An army of doctors were making their rounds this morning. The most important round of the week I guess, because they got to find out who had got better, who had got worse, who was new and if anyone had popped their clogs. If anyone had, perhaps Friday should have been the most important round of the week. I had my questions ready when they got round to me. Six doctors stood around my bed including Dr. Snell, the consultant, Dr. Ng and Dr. Kumar, the S.H.O.s. The others, I guessed, were being shown the ropes. Hallamshire was a teaching hospital. If they weren't students it seemed a waste of NHS funds, and God knows I had already had more spent on me than I would ever pay in.

They checked me over and asked all the standard dinner party ice-breaker questions, such as: Vomiting much? Any blood in your stools? Diarrhoea? I shook my head. "Tip top", I said. Dr. Snell said he had been told of my request to return to the Royal, and he put his hands on his hips in an I'm-not-very-happy-about-it kind of way. "Once you start a course of treatment with us we like to see it through," he said as sternly as a man who isn't very stern could. "If you still want to pursue it we can see if it's possible but, obviously, it would have to be sooner rather than later." I was nodding a bit too much. I stopped nodding, realising it was my turn to say something, "Well I appreciate that. It's really just a case of it being easier for my family and my personal circumstances if I'm there." A woman to my far right that I hadn't even spotted chimed in that she had spoken to Alison this week who had said they were keen to get me back. Between us we seemed to win Dr. Snell over. It was agreed that the woman would telephone Alison that afternoon to discuss if and when they could co-opt me back. I thanked them and pressed on to the slightly more serious matter of my next question, which exact type of AML I had and what significance that had on my chances. "Well, you're in the standard risk category," he said. "We tend to deal in those terms rather than the exact type of the disease, as the treatment would be the same." I didn't feel satisfied and he saw it. "We know that you're in standard risk so we know it's not one of the nasties." He went on, "You have about a 50 per cent chance of putting this behind you." My face didn't move, but suddenly I was looking somewhere past Dr. Snell. Those were at least 20 per cent lower odds than I had previously heard. I had just had 20 per cent knocked off my chances, and I felt like it. My stomach twisted. "But, you know, given your age, I'd say ... how old are you?" "25." His eyes went upwards, as if he was doing a sum. Maybe he was. "I'd say you have a touch better chance. You know 50...something maybe. I nodded solemnly; resignedly realising it didn't change one iota how I felt about everything. He could have told me I had a 15 per cent chance and it wouldn't change my attitude. Anyone who told me that, fuck them, no offence, I'd be the fifteenth through the door, I'd make it.

Dr. Snell looked as though he'd forgotten something. He put a hand to the side of his head. "Mr. Woolley, tell me, do you remember being told if you have what we call the 'Flt3' mutation?" I knew what he meant. I was tested for it at Chesterfield. Those with it are treated with an additional drug during course 1 of chemo. I didn't have it. "Oh, that's good," Dr. Snell said. I sensed relief in his voice. "Those with it don't tend to do as well. About 15 per cent or so is the success rate." My eyebrows bounced off the ceiling. I had no idea so much was riding on that test. Dr. Strong had always talked about Flt3 in very casual terms and when I was told I didn't have it, it was something of an afterthought. I realised it was probably not wise to tell every patient the numbers beforehand but I wanted at least to know I should have been celebrating not being a Flt3-er. The doctors left me to mull over those little pearlers.

I looked across at Brian, the new bloke on the ward. My eaves dropping had already told me he had Hodgkin's Lymphoma and shadows on the lungs. He wore an oxygen mask or a nebuliser most of the time and could hardly catch his breath to speak. I knew he was an ex-smoker and I wondered how much that affected the level of sympathy he got. He seemed a nice enough chap, but I wished he would turn down the volume on his TV from time to time. Occasionally I would see him cough up something black into a cup. I thought how awful it must be to have lung disease, the discomfort so constant. I tried to never look at those around me and think "Hey, at least I haven't got what you've got." That's not quite the point. But I would look around and see such people, and others, who couldn't walk, couldn't speak, couldn't stand, couldn't hear, and allow a sort of gratitude to replenish me. Never must I get down about what I couldn't do. Only celebrate what I could. I was the healthiest and most mobile person on the ward. Hell, if we'd held our own Olympics I'd have cleaned up.

I looked over at my table and caught sight of a rogue penny. 50/50 ah? I considered not doing it, all the time staring at the coin, knowing I would. I placed the penny on the top of my thumb, with the nail coiled under my index finger. I took a breath. Tails I live, heads I die.

I flipped the coin, caught it and slapped it on the back of my left hand. In that moment I had the same belief in this coin toss as I did in myself. I already knew. The penny had been on my table for days. I didn't know where it had come from. Now it seemed the most natural thing that it was waiting to prove something to me. I slowly lifted my right hand. It was a tail. I nodded. QED.

Tuesday June 17 2008. Course 2: Day 9.

I was in the shower when I felt the lump. A little knot on my left testicle. I'd always been proactive in checking because I always had a fear of something happening there which bordered on paranoia. A few times in the past I had thought I'd found a lump before realising I was mistaken. This time was different. There was no mistaking it. I felt my blood pump harder as I checked again. I kept thinking, "Come on. Now this too? Is someone taking the piss?" I dried off and dressed, went back to my bed and phoned Mary. I wanted her to say: "Don't be daft. Nothing to worry about. Forget it." She didn't. She said I was scaring her and I needed to tell someone straight away. Of course she was right. I should know how important being proactive was. Health was too precious to leave to chance. My problem wasn't with the inevitable examinations, surely it was worse for the examiner, it was with being told there was something wrong. I had a flashback to that free-falling moment when Mary told me I had leukaemia. My only comfort coming from the fact, I thought I might still be dreaming. I didn't know what the implications were if it was a tumour. Did it mean the cancer had spread, taken hold somewhere else? I didn't know if that was likely or even possible, but negative thoughts began creeping in like dark margins on my sight. The doctors were on their rounds, so I would have the perfect opportunity to raise the issue. While they zigzagged from bed to bed in bay to bay I lay there unable to do or think anything else, unwilling to even lose myself in a newspaper. When Dr. Ng came to see me with just one junior doctor, I was relieved the rest of the circus wasn't with her. We talked about the usual things first before I dropped the ball. She looked a little surprised, coming as this revelation had from left-field. "I will ask Dr. Kumar to examine you," she said, on her way out.

I nervously paced up and down beside my bed, which was really only long enough for one pace each way. I wondered on the etiquette of such things, I imagined that already being stripped to the waist when the doctor came in would make me look too eager at best. Should I take the jeans off, though? Debatable. In the end Dr. Kumar found me fully clothed. He had a slightly confused look on his face, and said only: "Er, a lump?" "Yes" I said. "I first noticed it this morning." "Any pain or discomfort with it? Any swelling?" "No, not that I've noticed." He nodded, which I saw as my signal to get my balls out. These were strange times. I lay on the bed and Dr. Kumar's gloved hands began examining me like a judge on the vegetable stall at a church fete. His eyes were somewhere far away as he worked. I didn't really know what to do with my hands. "There is definitely something there," he said, tearing my thoughts back from mild embarrassment to fear. "But I don't think it's anything to worry about. I think it's probably physiological rather than a ..." He paused, not wanting to say the word. I mentally filled in the word 'tumour' like some horribly graphic game of *Blankety Blank*. As though thinking the word and not saying it was any better. He snapped off his gloves. "If it was me, I wouldn't be worried, but I will ask for you to see a urologist, as I'm not an expert in this."

Dr. Kumar said it should not delay my switch to Chesterfield, as I could always see one of the specialists there. Even though I was now dressed the doctor was still staring at my groin as he spoke. I took heart from what he said, but by his own admission he was not a specialist in these matters, so until I had the word from them I wasn't going to be able to stop worrying. Dr. Kumar told me later I was going to have an ultrasound scan, the same device they use to spy on babies in the womb. I wondered if they could tell me if the lump was a boy or a girl, but mentally noted not to say that to the urologist. It sounded like one of those jokes you think is original but they've heard a million times. It was now a case of waiting.

William was looking worse by the day. Last night he had fallen badly. I looked up from my book to see him tumble over his Zimmer frame and against the window ledge, crumpling into a heap on the floor. I pulled the emergency buzzer and all the team came running in to help. The buzzers were usually false alarms and when they were you could laugh at the gaggle of nurses running in a line minus the Benny Hill theme tune. This was no false alarm, however, and William had cut his face and neck and hurt his side. I had seen him shuffling on his frame towards nowhere. When doctors asked him what he'd been doing, he said someone had called his name "out there", and pointed to the window. We were five floors up. I'd seen it in him all the previous day, he couldn't seem to summon any strength or lucidity. In fact, all around me seemed to be deteriorating. George was sleeping more and more, even though his sense of humour occasionally broke through. One day Austin, one of the nurses, and I were discussing footballers' salaries. Austin said to George: "Would you fancy £120k a week George?" George paused there, blinking, and neither of us expected him to answer. "I'd do it for £115k," he said. "But I'd have to cut back on a few luxuries."

Brian meanwhile was going downhill fast. The oxygen level in his blood which should be 100%, was down around 72%, and he just couldn't get his breath. During the day, as I waited to see the urologist, I saw them hook him up to some industrial breathing equipment, put in a catheter and summon a nurse from the High Dependency Unit. Before long, he was shipped off wholesale. The way he looked when they moved him out of the bay, Mary and I both feared he wouldn't make it through the night. We wished his wife good luck. Hospitals can be the most inspiring or soul-destroying places. Yes, there was a great deal of suffering, but there was also compassion, warmth and love in evidence everywhere you looked. At times like these though, seeing what was happening to Brian, George and William, as well as worrying about what my scan would reveal, made it too much. The feel of the ward could be oppressive, and sometimes I needed to get off it, and have a shot of normality.

But today I was waiting for news from the ward at Chesterfield as well as to be summoned by the urologist. The hours were ticking by and Mary and I were getting fraught with not knowing. We ended up taking our frustrations out on each other. We fell out a couple of times and Mary was clearly shaken by the events of the day. In the end I spoke to the charge nurse about whether I was likely to get closure on either of the things for which we were waiting. He phoned the urology department who confirmed I would not be seen that day. Then he phoned Durrant Ward and learned it was closed yet again because of C-diff. The outbreak they thought was under control clearly hadn't been. I knew then I would be finishing my course at Sheffield. I would not pin my hopes on Chesterfield again. Although I knew they wanted to have me back and were doing all they could to contain the outbreak, there was no chance of them stamping it out soon enough. I would be foolish to go back until they were proven to be long rid of it. "Well what now?" Mary asked me. I shrugged and looked out of the window. "I fancy a cheese burger."

Wednesday June 18 2008. Course 2: Day 10.

I was glad to be rid of the nausea and vomiting the chemo drugs induced, but without the doses at 10 a.m. and 10 p.m. to punctuate the days, they felt strangely hollow. I would look to fill up each moment with something, I get an itch when I'm idle, but I felt forever like a man who enters a room and freezes because he can't remember why he went in. I always felt like there was something else I should be doing, could be doing but never seemed able to find it and settle. Today I was particularly lacking in attention span as I waited to hear about my ultrasound. Dr. Kumar had been confident I was okay but I still felt apprehensive, there was something growing where it should definitely not be growing and that is never good as far as I was concerned.

I saw Dr. Kumar again in the morning and we exchanged the sly nod of two men, who have been far too intimate. When he saw me on his rounds we talked about what was to come. My counts were coming down nicely so I could expect to start feeling flat within a couple of days. Much later on, at around Day 25, I should start to pick up, before being discharged on Day 28. That was 18 days from now, and I had to bounce off the bottom to reach that ceiling. It seemed the second course of chemo could be much more predictable than the first, and I found it useful to be given a really clear picture. Eighteen days to get through. We talked briefly about infections, which I felt certain to get, being on the ward this time. My immune system would be zero so I was guaranteed to pick things up, at which point I would be given antibiotics to combat it. Sometimes, at Chesterfield, they took blood cultures to try and find what the infection was and which antibiotic would be most effective. Very few people get through a course without an infection but there was no harm in trying to be one of the few. I needed to be proactive with my mouth washing and keep clean. This time I was sharing bathrooms though so the odds were really stacked against me.

I had just finished dinner when I was brought one of those charming backward surgical gowns and told I had half an hour before they would come to fetch me for the ultrasound. I turned the gown over a full three times before I figured out the entrance. Again I wondered on the boxer short etiquette, opting to keep them on. I sat and shivered in the draught, considering how many bizarre procedures I was intent on going through during my illness: bone marrow biopsy, Hickman line installation, sperm cryogenics, rectal exam and, now, testicular ultrasound. I tried to envisage a situation where such a list of experiences might be beneficial, perhaps some game of health care *Top Trumps*, but thought the only good I could draw would be my friends' amusement at my anecdotes. They would be dearly-bought laughs I hoped they would appreciate.

Before too long I was being wheeled, bald headed and besmocked, down to the ultrasound department, probably looking every inch a cancer victim to those who passed by. The porter left me in a kind of holding area alongside a few others on beds and wheelchairs. Some I could guess what they were having scanned, others not. I could tell they were probably playing the same game with me. When my turn came, I was disappointed to have a pretty gormless-looking lad of my age escort me in. I had foolishly thought a doctor would carry out the scan and give an opinion there and then. As it was, Alan, for he looked like an Alan, would wield the probe and take some snaps for his superior to report back on. I was asked to drop 'em and lie on the bed while Alan put on some romantic mood-lighting. I was half expecting Rod Stewart tunes to click on to get me in the mood further. Alan sniffed loudly and informed me he was going to "scan the testes", which was a relief seeing as that's why I was there. If he had tried to probe my womb we would have fallen out. He pulled out a squeezy tube of gel lubricant, which I imagined he would carry in a holster if they let him and squidged it liberally over the end of the probe. It resembled one of those hand held bar code scanners, only smothered in lube. Alan sniffed again. "This will feel cold," he said, making contact. I tried to crane my neck and see the screen, but wasn't best placed to see anything other than vague shapes in shades of grey, so I sat back. After a minute he switched to the side in question, pausing to reapply the gel. I could hear him zooming in and out and taking stills. "Any lumps or bumps?" he asked. I paused, wondering if he had even been made aware of why I was there. "Erm, yes," I said. "Can you find it for me?" I did, and he began probing again and snapping pictures. I tried again to catch sight of the screen and the imposter in my nut sack. But it was already over. Alan took something from the computer, some disk or memory device, and made for the door, telling me a porter would escort me up to G-floor. "What happens now?" I got in before he left. "We send it up to your ward and the doctors will let you know." I wasn't sure what "it" he was referring to. I waited a moment, quietly in that room, listening to the gentle hum of the ultrasound machine, and asked myself how I'd got here, how my life had changed. So much, so quickly.

Back on the ward, Mary was waiting for me. The ward seemed busy today, thronging with patients, visitors and doctors all bouncing around off one another. There was even a group of army cadets standing around blocking the main thoroughfare for whatever reason. I had a pounding headache, which I put down to my counts, and the activity just increased the pressure on my head. A new patient had been moved in opposite me. Dennis was his name and rudeness was his game. I marvelled at the way he addressed staff, with everything from a whistle to, once, a bark. Please and thank you did not appear to be in his vocabulary. As far as I could tell there was little wrong with him, yet he attempted nothing by himself. He was trigger-happy with the buzzer and kept it within easy reach at all times. It was inevitable, I supposed, that I would meet patients I didn't like occasionally. Just because people are old and sick doesn't mean they can't be arseholes. If Dennis got bored he would just stare at me, perhaps waiting for me to spring out of bed and entertain him like his personal court jester. Occasionally I would stare back, thinking he would get the hint and look at something else: he would not. The longest I managed was about 10 seconds' worth of his icy, unblinking stare before I looked away first, slightly afraid of what he may do to me as I slept, if he could be arsed to get out of bed, that is.

While Dennis, who didn't appear too badly off, could grumble about everything, George, a gentle soul, was very little trouble to anyone. He was in his sixties, a passionate *Blades* fan with a kind smile. He had six months to live, I had learned. Today, George was confused. Several times during the day he had called his wife's name, Jane. It was outside visiting hours and she wasn't there. Each time I would get up and ask a nurse to go and help him with whatever it was he needed. Each time I would see him realise where he was, and a little bit more of his soul would drain away. Later in the day I looked up and George was reaching a hand towards me asking me to help him. I should have fetched a nurse but it felt like he was asking me to do it, and that would be the wrong thing to do. George was half way to sitting up, his legs draped over the side of the bed. I took his hand and he gripped it tightly. He was a big man and I knew it hurt for him to move. He had a suspected tumour on his spine for which he would have radiotherapy, among his other problems. "Help me sit," he said. I pulled lightly against him, not wanting to move him too fast. I kept my arm firm for him to pull against me and soon he was red in the face and out of breath but upright. I asked if he was okay. He looked at me and I wasn't sure he knew who I was, but he nodded. Jane, his wife, appeared soon after. Mary had been talking to her in the corridor and learned that they had been married only five years, having both lost their former partners, his to breast cancer and hers to a brain tumour.

For some reason I thought of a piece I'd seen in the paper that day. It had a line-up of photographs of men; the pictures all aged—depicted were the ten most wanted Nazi war criminals. With each there was information on where they were thought to be hiding out under assumed names. Each man in his 90s, living the life they deprived of so many. There seemed little fairness left in the world.

George was telling Jane something. "My wife's going to play hell," he said. "I'm your wife George. Why would I play hell with you?" "For coming out dressed like this" he gestured at himself. She put a hand on his shoulder and I could hear the tears in her voice. "George, where do you think you are?" He looked her in the eye as though offended she was asking. "I'm on the playing fields," he said. Jane turned away and cried out, before composing herself "No, George, you're in hospital. You're not very well." He looked at his lap, crestfallen. I turned away. Mary's eyes were brimming over. "I'm sorry," George said. "I'm going daft aren't I?"

That night I had a dream. I dreamed that I and four friends were attempting to cross the English Channel on surf boards. For whatever reason, the water was green and warm as we paddled out from the beach happily. When we got so far, we spotted a wave coming towards us. It grew and grew until it was towering, roaring like a gale, ten storeys high. The sky turned black, the water icy cold. Before it hit us, I looked across at my friends and saw their faces had changed. They were not my friends at all. I tried to take a breath as the wave crashed, but inhaled only water, and was buried under the storm.

Thursday June 19 2008. Course 2: Day 11.

A man passed me in the corridor, and we said hello, each of us carrying towels under our arms. I hadn't seen him before on the ward. He looked in his early 30s and had the tell-tale chemo-chic hairstyle. He looked as though he might have leukaemia, I considered, and thought that, by the 50/50 rule, one of us wouldn't make it. The thought hung there for a moment longer than I would like, lingering after I tried to forget it. My philosophy thus far had been not to think on things too deeply, or for too long. It seemed to me there was little to be gained from thinking myself into a hole. But I had a fair bit on my plate at that time. I had leukaemia of course, that was a shame, I had a lump in an unfortunate place, the stress of a wedding in 12 weeks time and to top it all, a leaky roof.

By now one of the roofers had come back to us and given a very grim picture of things up top. Our roof, it seemed, had been patched up by cowboys and the result was a horror show. Tiles were wedged in gaps, other spaces were left wide open and the materials used were unsuitable. The roofer was amazed we only had the one leak. Bottom line: repairs £1K, new roof £4K. It may as well be £40K, we didn't have it, couldn't borrow it. Our credit had been stretched to the limit when we bought the house the previous year, and the U.K. was now in the grip of an economic slowdown. The timing was impeccable. All the money we had was tied up in the wedding other than the cash raised for us at the FA Cup Final event, in *the Woolley Hat Fund*. Mary and I discussed it and agreed that to spend the money on roof repairs went against the spirit in which it was raised. We felt it was there to allow the two of us to do something life-changing after this was over. I was old enough to know that when you get a bit of money in this life, something will immediately surface and speak for it. We were awaiting a couple more quotations for the roof, but we had a ballpark figure for the damage. Whatever happened next, we would have to make do for a while with the blue bags I had stuffed in the hole. I made a conscious effort to put the roof to the back of my mind being as it was, the least of my problems and as I could do nothing about it at present.

Then, just as I had done so, the vacuum was filled with another problem, as though there was some sort of cosmic osmosis at work. I overheard two of the sisters as they changed shift, saying that there was something of a diarrhoea outbreak. It would seem that everyone in one of the bays, along with a handful of others, had the runs. My own episode had long come to an end but I wondered if some bug was stalking me, across two hospitals and in different counties. There was no indication this was C-diff but that was my fear, the worst case scenario. But even if it wasn't it was an infection I would have to contend with, having no immune system. The ward had shared patient toilets and those would be where it spread. I had already developed something of an obsession with washing my hands, so much so that the alcohol hand wash was starting to burn holes on the backs of my fingers. I touched nothing I didn't have to. This regime would stand me in good stead as I made a bid to get through this chemo without an infection, but some of it was out of my control. I could easily fall prone to an infection that was previously dormant in my own body. It was as much luck as anything else, just like the success of the treatment, it seemed.

Suddenly the curtain was whipped around my bed and the full complement of doctors filed in like children who'd heard the bell for the end of break time. Dr Snell took the space to my left hand, as always wearing a suit that looked too big for him. He carried the easy confidence of a man who explains immensely complicated things to people who shun the complicated, and even use of the word 'immensely'. I wanted to cut the pleasantries and go straight for the balls, so to speak. Did I have anything to worry about? Would I be known from now on as Johnny Two-cancers? Had my leukaemia manifested itself and this was only the first of many complications? "We've had the results from the urologist," Dr. Snell said. My heart was pumping so hard I swear they could all hear it. "It's a cyst, and nothing at all to worry about." I let out my breath in a quick, noisy rasp, so that the doctors looked up from their clipboards; and I felt elation and embarrassment in equal measure. I sat back in a futile attempt to regain the cool I had just blown out of my mouth. "That's great," I said. "That's a relief." He moved on swiftly to my main problem and scanned my notes. I exchanged a glance with Dr. Kumar, thinking it must have been a relief for him too; having gone to great lengths to reassure me it was nothing. I considered that now that problem was torpedoed, what might fill its space, under my hastily-conceived cosmic osmosis theory. Another problem? An opportunity would be nice. Maybe I could fill it with jelly babies, I didn't really understand it, and it was my theory. I realised I wasn't listening to the people who were being paid to save my life and thought I'd better snap out of it. We discussed how I was feeling, to which my reply was, "suspiciously well." It was true. I felt good, but knew the pain was coming, like a man walking blind-fold towards the cliff edge. My counts were low, I knew that, but the sun was shining and who knew?

I thought back to the day before I was admitted to hospital. My counts were through the floor, dangerously low. If I'd cut myself badly I would have bled to death. In all fairness I should have been flat out on the floor, where was I? In the pub, blissfully unaware anything was wrong. I did wonder why I had a green face, but other than that I was living, working, eating and doing everything that people without leukaemia do.

I had the urge to dip my toe back into the waters of normality so when my friend, Christian, and Mary arrived; I decided to sneak out for a couple of hours. We drove into town and went for something to eat in a pub. The place was empty, which was one of the criteria for me. I went to the bar to order our food and was met by a stoney-faced bulk of muscle behind the pumps. Perhaps he was a bouncer who'd got lost. "I'd like to order some food please," I smiled. "I.D. please," he said, face hardly moving. I frowned. "No, we're not drinking; I'd just like to order some food." He was not amused. "We have a Challenge 25 policy. Anybody who looks under 25 has to show I.D., some pubs have a Challenge 21, we have a Challenge 25." I think I was supposed to be in some way impressed by this. I persevered. "Mate, I'm only ordering food. I don't have my wallet with me. I am 25 years old." The bulky barman closed his eyes, effecting the impression of someone who is so bored he cannot even stay awake. "I need to see something with D.o.B. on it. I felt the anger rising to a ball in my throat, which threatened to turn itself into words I'd regret. I turned around and walked away from the over-inflated meathead. They say steroids make you grumpy. I swallowed my rage and we left. Just as we got outside we walked into the entire line-up of the band Boyzone on the street. All in all, a very bizarre two-and-a-half minutes. Only later in the day did I realise I was wearing my hospital bracelet the whole time, which is emblazoned with my date of birth. I half considered going back.

Friday June 20 2008. Course 2. Day 12.

The hospital wants you to be awake. It stirs at around 6 a.m., and the volume and intensity rises until you do. It behaves like a child jumping on your bed on Christmas morning; only

Christmas comes 365 times a year. Today I am tired but I've no chance of any sleep. Others around me, namely George and Dennis, can and do sleep during the day, but they were the types to wake up and find they'd missed an air raid. The choice made for me; I got up and began the game of strategy that is getting a shower. There were three on the ward but bagging one took skill and aggression, you had to spot your opening and dash for it. If you ploughed down an old lady with her beach towel and Marks & Spencer wash bag, so be it. Collateral damage. The games were not aided by the fact that occasionally one or more of the showers would be closed for variable issues with plumbing. Other times I would open the door to find a used bedpan awaiting collection from the floor. The door kind of closes itself when you see that. I managed to get one eventually and when I padded back to my bed in my slippers, Vanessa was waiting to see me. Vanessa liaised with patients to make sure they had everything they needed and the boredom wouldn't make them eat their own thumbs. I still had mine for now. We had a chat about how things were going, and how I felt mentally.

Across from me Dennis pressed his buzzer for the tenth time that morning. I wondered if I could attach the wire to him somehow so he got shocked every time he pressed it. I looked back at Vanessa. She was telling me about the new Haematology Ward which was being built higher up the concrete dragon on P-floor. Where we were now, Ward G-2, was a temporary base while the swanky new ward was finished. It would have new facilities for younger people to make their stay less hellish, such as computers and games, etc. "How old are you Richard?" she asked. "I'm 25," I said. She pursed her lips, as though I'd given an incorrect answer. I thought about dropping it down a bit. 16 may be. "The programme is meant to cater for people up to 24. You don't qualify as a young person." That was it then, I thought, the exact moment my youth ended and I became a grown-up. She was mulling it over, perhaps imagining some scenario in which the SAS might have to raid the computer room on intelligence an adult was in there. "When was your birthday?" "April," I said, stifling a laugh at the silly bureaucracy of it all. Her eyes softened a little. "Oh that's okay. You're only just 25." I thought the SAS would see it that way too. "When is this new unit going to be finished?" Her eyes darted quickly to the right, as though I'd asked a question that would compromise her. "Well," she paused. "It was supposed to be in the middle of July but they've told us they're three weeks behind. At least." I saw where this was going. "My office is still up there. It's a mess still at the moment. They've got to finish it then clean it, paint it and clean it again, then move everything back in." As if for finality, she added: "The absolute deadline is October." I blinked, wondering why we were even having this conversation now. If that was the time scale, I prayed I would never see the place, swanky or not.

We moved on to the subject of the wedding and I asked if I might be able to sit down with Dr. Snell sometime soon to discuss the issue. I didn't know if the wedding date was still in any way feasible or if we should move either the date itself or delay my last treatment. Vanessa agreed, but recommended we wait until after this treatment, when we would have an idea of how quickly I recovered. That sounded fair to me. As she packed up her things, Vanessa asked: "How are you and your fiancée coping financially?" Now there was a can of worms. "We're struggling a bit," I said. Mary had spent £80 on petrol that week alone, not to mention the parking fees, probably upwards of £25. Mary was off work, we were only getting a flat rate, minus extras for unsociable hours, so we were down a couple of hundred quid a month. It wasn't that rosy, all in all, not with any savings we had spoken for in the wedding budget. "You could consider applying for a grant towards your expenses," Vanessa said. My first reaction was that this was a good idea. I did have cancer, and there were measures in place to help people like me. I said I would discuss it with Mary later.

When we did talk it over, we both agreed not to apply. The awarding body was MacMillan Nurses, who offer palliative care to victims of cancer. From what little I knew of their work, they did a fantastic job on stretched resources. There would be cases much more pressing than ours and we didn't even want to waste their time by putting in our application. We'd get by, one way or another. I told Mary if things got too bad, I'd sell my body. She laughed a little too hard.

As we sat talking, Dr. Kumar came over to me looking tense. Minutes earlier I had walked past him as he conversed with Drs. Snell and Ng. From the way they looked at me and said hello, I had the distinct impression the case they were discussing was my own. It turned out I was right. Dr. Kumar cleared his throat and began. "Richard, I've just spoken to the Royal Hospital in Chesterfield and they have a bed for you." I knew this would happen. For all the respect and gratitude I owed the doctors there, their timing was shit. I'd been saying all week that if they offered me a bed at this late stage I would turn them down flat. Now the offer was on the table and I was tempted. "Dr. Snell is not all together happy with the idea but he doesn't want to stand in your way if you want to go." I looked at Mary and we both sighed. I now had neutrophil levels, my body's defence against infection, of 0.1, meaning I was wide open to catching anything and everything. My platelets, too, were rock bottom, so strictly speaking, I shouldn't be moved. If I went, I might arrive at Chesterfield and find that the C-diff bug flared up again immediately. I was now settled at Sheffield, knew where I was with the doctors and, frankly, would feel downright rude if I walked out now. I knew all this, so why did part of me still want to go? I felt there was a subtle tug-of-war between the hospitals over me, born of each one's duty of care. They both felt I was their patient. Chesterfield, I thought, felt guilty enough over what had gone on before that they were willing to have me back even though the timing was all wrong. Sheffield held all the cards but was willing to let me go if I thought that was best for my care. There would be advantages if I went, namely isolation and more flexible visiting hours. Mary looked me in the eye and I knew there was only one choice I could make. "I think it's best that I stay here." Dr. Kumar didn't smile but nodded. "I think that's the right thing," he said. "I will ring them and cancel the bed."

Saturday June 21 2008. Course 2: Day 13.

My proactive attitude towards hygiene had officially lurched off into obsession. I was washing my hands every half hour or so, then using the alcohol hand-rub any time I touched anything. I rinsed my mouth out with the antibacterial mouthwash at least four times a day or straight away if someone breathed on me or I got a whiff of a bad smell. I held paper towels to open the door in the bathroom or to touch the light switch. I held my breath when people came near to me. Part of me even wanted to withdraw when Mary got too close. She sensed this and, while it must have been a little upsetting, she respected my feelings on it. I didn't feel I was doing it compulsively; my determination not to get sick had simply morphed into a fear of getting sick. The episodes in which I was ill during my first course were dreadful and not easily forgotten. I was terrified of going back there. I was terrified of germs. If I had to live like a poor man's Howard Hughes for a while then I would do it gladly. I likened my predicament to my leaky roof. Occasionally, when the immune system is normal, the odd leak might get through. Right then it was like I had no roof at all. I was not even in isolation this time round, dozens of people trouped in and out of my bay every day. But being shut away hadn't prevented me getting sick last time, so it offered no guarantees. All I could do was keep away from people as much as possible and keep my guard up. My counts were now rock bottom, and not just for my immune system. Both my red blood cells and platelets were all but killed off by the chemo.

On a trip to the bathroom, a nurse stopped me to ask if I would be shaving that day. "Am I making the place look scruffy?" I asked. Days earlier, the same nurse had helped me open one of those infernally-well shrink wrapped packs of shaving razor heads. She had warned me then that, while my counts were down, they didn't like patients using razors. Today I was expressly banned from shaving. My platelets, which help the blood to clot, were at a level of six, somewhere up around 160 being normal. I was going to need some by transfusion. Either that or I would start to look like my head was upside down

Sunday June 22 2008. Course 2: Day 14.

For the second day I woke up with a blinding headache. It was noisy and the bustle of the ward felt like it was pressuring my head from all sides. This presented a problem in that most of the painkillers on offer disagreed with my sanity. Paracetamol was a safe bet but the doctors were reluctant to give it to me as it masked a temperature, the first indicator of infection. In the end I persuaded them to give me paracetamol, which was enough to take the edge of the headache though was hardly the strongest thing on the market.

I had hardly slept thanks to Dennis' constant coughing, which he did in the most vile way, and relentless buzzer-pushing. He had also wet his bed after trying to fill one of the urine bottles while lying down, being too lazy to sit up, which everyone knew he was more than capable of doing. The thing that unsettled me most about the man was the fact he never did anything to pass the time. Whereas I felt driven to fill up every minute with reading, writing, TV or music; Dennis would just lie there, winding down the clock impervious to boredom. His only amusement came from ordering people to do things, which wasn't limited to nursing staff, visitors and even other patients were asked to pass him a urine bottle, pour him a drink or countless other things he was capable of doing himself. If he had his fill of that, he could also resort to staring at me, which he did for at least a couple of hours each day. He was due to be sent home soon and I was looking forward to seeing the back of him, especially after I overheard that he too had diarrhoea.

The doctors said I was due for a unit of blood that day, to boost my flagging haemoglobin counts. My neutrophils were 0.0, this was officially no roof territory. I was praying and pleading with every fibre for sunshine. I asked Dr. Snell if it was customary to give patients a GCSF injection at this stage. He looked a little surprised; I had never sprung research on him before. GCSF was a growth hormone, the same used ahead of a stem cell harvesting. It stimulates the bone marrow into working extra hard to get the body back on track. "The problem is," Dr. Snell said, "that it's quite an artificial result. When we stop giving the injections all the counts go down again and it's disappointing for everyone." He cupped each hand which protruded from a baggy sleeve. "We don't tend to use it unless we've gone a long time without satisfactory movement in the counts." I nodded, weighing up where this new piece of information left me. I asked if I was going to get any antibiotics as a precaution. I wondered if he could tell I was scared. He shook his head, "No, we don't do that." But he went on; perhaps sensing I wanted some help: "Look, everything is looking good so far. You're a young lad who should be able to bounce back quickly. Did you recover quickly last time?" "No," I said, and everyone laughed spontaneously. It wasn't pitched as a joke. "Okay, so it may take a little longer, but the longer you can keep free of infection, that will help your body return to normal quicker."

Everyone always talked about infections as a certainty when your counts are rock bottom. But the odd few must get through. I was odd; I could give an odd duo the third leg of their tripod of oddness. I was foolish enough to disclose this ambition to Sharon, one of many excellent nurses on the ward. She wished me luck with it and then we got talking about each of our weddings which, it turned out, were on precisely the same day, only hers was in Las Vegas. "What made you choose there?" I asked. "Well I don't like a fuss, so ..." "So you chose Las Vegas? Have you not seen the brochure?" As we talked I began wondering if I should have kept quiet about my determination to get through this with no infection. It was an unspoken ambition of everyone who played the game, I supposed, but I was actively seeking to prove it was possible. Now I'd gone and said it.

Later on in the night Sharon dropped in a leaflet on The Willow Trust, the charity set up by former Arsenal and Scotland goalkeeper, Bob Wilson, following the death of his daughter, Anna, to cancer. The charity essentially offers big days out for young people with terminal or serious illnesses. The leaflet showed pictures of smiling faces, most of whom I couldn't tell were 'ill'. They enjoyed day trips with their friends to a show or to a sporting event. The Trust looked like a wonderful cause, but, again, I didn't feel comfortable taking any money out of it. We had *the Woolley Hat Fund* to use, unlike the young people in the leaflet. What was more; the dichotomy of its cheery tone and grim subject matter hit me like a jab in the ribs. Here was someone else lumping in my disorder with others considered 'life-threatening'. I started crying, for the first time in what felt like weeks, though I couldn't tell why.

Monday June 23 2008. Course 2: Day 15.

I'd spiked a temperature in the night and it was steadily rising. This was it. The signs were that I had an infection. Rising temperature, coupled with shivering and feeling tired all pointed that way, but I wasn't going to believe it until that temperature went above 38.8 degrees. If my determination hadn't worked, perhaps trusty old denial might do the trick. But silently both Mary and I were distraught. Things had been so good up until that point, and I had fashioned a fools dream it could always be that way. The speed at which the doctors moved the next day went beyond what I'd expected. I would be given a course of several IV antibiotics to halt the charge of it, but it seemed a lot of my levels were low as well. I needed potassium, tablets shaped like a baked bean, and magnesium. The only thing I remembered of that element from school was stealing strips of it from the Chemistry Lab to burn on the playing field. We would come around and watch it glow a brilliant white, fascinated as little boys are by fire. The tablet was huge and white, far too big to be swallowed. "You can chew it," a nurse said helpfully. "Yeah, but what does it taste like?" "I dunno. Never 'ad one 'ave I?" She was an astute girl. It was like chewing chalk and dust. All the saliva immediately soaked into it and I got far more of it stuck round my teeth than I could swallow. Eventually after adding about half a pint of water I created a paste that went down lovely. Another life experience ticked off.

By this point I was beginning to feel ill and absolutely exhausted. I could barely keep my eyes open for more than a few seconds. In some small way that was a pleasure. Just a day earlier I had lain there, blood boiling as Dennis snored loudly in the afternoon. The previous night he had kept me awake with his vile coughing, hocking and retching. Now he soundly slept while I could not. Only for so long could I stand it. On my way to the sink in our bay, which was conveniently next to Dennis' bed, I 'accidentally' gave the metal bin en route a thunderous kick. A few people looked up from the corridor with bemused faces and a start; I just carried on my path to the sink, trying not to give away my limp. I stole a glance back over my shoulder at Dennis, the ogre had not even stirred. I pondered all the messy execution methods at my disposal as I rigorously brushed my teeth, then thought I should probably let the old boy off. My homicidal streak was only because I was dog-tired myself. That and nauseous.

I'd hoped I might be beyond the vomiting and the non-eating. Now when the meals were being delivered my stomach would swill its contents around like the bitter dregs of a once great pint. I would freeze when I heard the trolley. The sound of it was enough. Sometimes I would appease my stomach and just decline the meal; sometimes I would let them leave it. I had to have the spittoon tray right by me in any case. I always liked that such a charmingly archaic instrument was still being put to good use, albeit in a not very hard wearing cardboard form. I suppose it just sounded more civilised than shouting for a vomit-tray.

The doctors did their tests to try and identify the route of the infection. I knew this was harder said than done, since when, at Chesterfield, to my knowledge, they didn't find the cause of any of the infections I had. They did cure them however with an antibiotics splatter-gun, the same approach that would be employed here. I fully expected I would get back the red full body rash as a reaction to one of them. I didn't know which one had caused it, as I was on a few at any given time. I remember Dr. Cowdrey writing down which one he thought it probably was, but the several doctors and nurses I repeated this to looked mystified. One of them said: "We wouldn't have your notes from Chesterfield. We only have our notes." I was flabbergasted, genuinely making a little 'o' with my mouth. Surely it would have been beneficial to my case to have insight from my doctors, rather than what I could tell them? I mentioned someone might phone up Chesterfield and ask to be informed which drug they had down as the allergy. They laughed it off and said something about "never getting hold of the right person before we've given it to you anyway." Some of the old problems were returning too. I was constipated, as a result of the antibiotics, which made my stomach rock-solid. My backside was also sore again, making it difficult to get comfortable or sit upright. I was peeing in fits and bursts again, and it was difficult to get the flow going sometimes. The result: many hobbles up and down the corridor with a drip stand to the toilet. Later an on-call doctor's phone rang. His ring tone was *the Ring of Fire*.

Tuesday June 24 2008. Course 2: Day 16.

George was sent for a dose of radiotherapy on his back to try and shrink a tumour on his spine which was restricting his movement. Then he was due to go home. He didn't want to be admitted ever again. We wished him and Jane all the luck in the world on what was, coincidentally, Jane's birthday. Dennis was sent home too but we never got chance to hold each other tightly on a windy platform. He slipped out while I was off having a chest X-ray to look for any infection. I was wheeled down on my bed and left to wait in the corridor by the same porter who ferried me for my ultrasound. I slept. I was doing a lot of that this week. When I woke a man with a kind, yet impossibly-square face led me in to a square room and pointed some very silly, heavy and expensive equipment at my chest (apparently I have a long one?) for ten minutes or so. Then he wheeled me back into the hall and I went back to sleep. I was now on a couple of painkillers for my headache, which showed no sign of abating, and these had quite pleasant hallucinatory effects when I closed my eyes. I could see anything from my hospital bed, I could be flying fast and low through a jungle canopy getting scratched by the trees, or watch four Japanese people I didn't know have dinner in a restaurant. Sometimes I could affect what was going on, other times not, but I had to admit it was fun.

Being asleep most of the day helped with feeling sick, but as my body clock caught up I began to feel the all too familiar slide towards the edge. My bloods revealed I was low on levels of potassium and magnesium still, so I was going to need drips for those, blood, platelets, antibiotics and lots of saline because my blood pressure kept getting low. I was very low on everything really, which, along with the infection made me understand the true meaning of 'curl up and die'. Once again the drugs had done funny things to my head. Instead of thinking of myself in terms of 'me', I was again thinking about myself in the third person. If I got out of bed in the night and saw my dressing gown on the chair on the other side, a normal person's inner-monologue might go something like: "Oh, I'm cold and it's right over there. I'll have to unplug the drip stand and walk round to fetch it." The one more common in my head was something like this: "The kid's made a basic error. He's making work for himself. He'll have to walk right over there, let's see if he falls over!"

Wednesday June 25 2008. Course 2: Day 17.

Just after breakfast we were told the ward was having a little switch-around. The catalyst for this, as far as I could gather, was an old lady who was in bad shape and needed to be moved closer to the centre of the ward. The logistics of this meant several people had to be moved, me being one, William another. Ordinarily I would not have minded, but I was feeling like refried fertiliser at that moment and minded about everything.

This new room smelled funny, had none of the personal TVs and was right at the end of the hall. William and I definitely seemed to have got the suckers' end of the bargain. Will didn't let it bother him though; he just sat there smiling with his big baggy features, like a monkey in a cardigan. The other residents of this bay were; a man who could happily while away hours, tuning through interrupted dirges of static on his radio. Then there was the nomad, Malcolm, who would spend the nights walking around. He had some serious health problems which had affected the curvature of his spine so he found it very difficult to get comfortable at night. That was as much as I could really take in at that moment because my head felt like it had one of those lightening orbs inside it. The headache was getting worse and the doctors agreed to send me for a CT scan. Another week, another two additions to my collection of procedures, I thought. I had been impressed by how freely the hospital departments worked together at the Hallamshire. If a test could identify something, if it could rule something out, then you would have it. If there were two drugs that were effective, you would have both. There wasn't the same mood at the Royal. That was all down to money, I knew. Budgets. The mood there was down-beat; staff were doing the best job they were allowed to do. They were stretched to their limits by understaffing, and penny-pinched back in their advances to meet costs. Sheffield was a University Hospital and its budgets must have been beyond the imaginings of their compatriots in Chesterfield. They would have settled for enough staff to do the job.

I pondered this between naps as I waited on a trolley outside the CT room. It had been the same porter yet again who had collected me. "Bloody 'ell mate!" He said. "You're getting your money's worth, aren't you!" The scan was over before I knew it. I had seen them on TV, people disappearing headlong on a butcher's tray into a pod which could scan their whole body in three dimensions. I was asked to lie on the slab and put my head in this block which made sure it wasn't going anywhere. Then I was slid into the darkness of its mouth and told I mustn't open my eyes, as though I may learn the secret that it's all just toilet rolls and Lego in there. Lasers shone on me. There was juddering. It was all very *Kraftwerk*.

Thursday – Saturday: June 26 – 28 2008. Course 2: Days 18 - 20.

I suffered days of being peppered by antibiotics which was almost worse than being ill. I was forever tethered to the kinky hat stand they hung endless drips from. Everything was given with huge bags of saline and I wondered how all this water they were pouring in my veins was supposed to know where to go. I still had diarrhoea and, with what my body had thrown at it in the past three weeks; I wasn't in the least bit surprised. My backside now felt like it'd had a week in the stocks and everyone'd had a pop at it. Despite slowly filling up like a balloon, I was finding it harder to pass water. My cinematic hallucinations had shrunk into cheap cartoons, predictable and nasty. And I still didn't want to eat. The combination of these things was twisting me and gnawing at me, like a need to get free from a box.

When the doctors came round I felt sure they would give me something for the diarrhoea and something to help with the waterworks. They would not. "Stupid weekend doctors,"I remember cursing when they left. They were not stupid; they merely got a 20 second précis of a patient's condition and then had to respond to their demands. Their number one priority is always to fob you off until Monday, when your doctor will have to deal with it. He did this to me not very subtly and he left knowing I wanted to chop his feet off. As long as his job was easier, who cares if someone had to be in agony for two days, right? I told him I'd woken up with really sore hips and all round that area was painful, as I'd retained masses of the water. He looked a little concerned, then recovered, discussing a scan for Monday. What a prince among men. He asked if I wanted the curtain pulling round on his way out. I said "Let the Monday staff do it." He skulked away and I was left there, doubled upon the bed, knowing I would have to go through two more days of this feeling, at the least.

Mary came at the start of visiting and found me just a bald sobbing wreck, with huge belly and swollen ankles. Maybe it was a premonition of married life she needed to see. It took her a long time to calm me down and to make me agree to try and ride it out. When your whole day revolves around piss and shit you've gone wrong.

As soon as visiting time was over, they told me I was being moved again, this time into a side room. The reason was to isolate me because of my diarrhoea, which I couldn't imagine getting any better now until my normal cell counts started coming back. As they wheeled me and my small collection of belongings up the hall, I realised this was just going to make things harder. On the ward I had the daily dramas of other people's lives, the distractions and annoyances of their behaviour and the simple stimulation of change to show the passage of time. In this room it was just going to be me, the duel between my thoughts once again, which were turning darker by the hour. I didn't want this move, in all honesty it scared me but I wasn't being offered a choice.

By that evening I was feeling really ill in about every different way. It was day 20 of my treatment. This period was the tipping point; the next few days should be the bridge that led out of the depths of it all. For now I was writhing around in that room, begging whoever would listen to make it stop. I had heard an account recently of an Irish sportsman's slog through chemotherapy. He'd said something like: "They make you feel so ill you wish you were dead." Though it hadn't taken me quite to that place yet, I knew exactly what he meant. It was clear now that I'd been kidding myself in believing I could make it through without an infection. It was possible, I was sure, but I had gone and convinced myself I would do it, no question. When I did not and was taken ill, I was left feeling angry and disappointed at myself. Had I let my guard down or taken a stupid risk, had I overdone it physically and worn myself down? The broken bottle walk was all the more painful for the shards of the ego.

Sunday June 29 2008. Course 2: Day 21.

I sweated so much during the night I had to ask the nurses to change the sheets twice. It must have really poured out of me. My nightmares were twisted and cruel, but somehow recognisable. I had dreamt of being visited by some kind of monkey, which sat calmly on the end of my bed. It fixed me with a stare and told me I needed to guess his name. "Why?" I asked. "Because this is why you're here. This is the game." I said I didn't know his name, couldn't guess. The monkey was suddenly angered and rattled the frame of my bed, telling me I needed to understand, and understand quickly. "I will be back in an hour," the monkey said, calmly now, and exited by whatever means it had come in. I was somewhere between sleep and consciousness, shivering and sweating, pleading for it all to stop, when the monkey returned. But he had grown. He was now the size of a man; and the bed frame rattled with a clunk when he leapt onto it. I lay there breathing and staring, too afraid to move. We both seemed to wait for the other to speak, and, for the longest time, neither of us did. Until I mustered: "How many chances do I have?" The ape was enraged, even before I'd finished asking, and he shook the bed with such a ferocity that I thought someone may hear. I hoped someone may come. It was silent again, and the ape waited for a name, freezing me with hollow eyes. I tried to think of something topical, something related to my treatment. That's what this was all about, wasn't it? The name of a piece of equipment or treatment? He must share a name with one of them. I thought of my central line, through which I received all my drugs intravenously. "Hickman," I faltered. "Is it Hickman?" The ape watched me through the darkness, and then slowly climbed down from the bed. "I will be back in an hour," he said. I sweated and turned, and for a while seemed to dream of other things, before finding myself back in my room, scanning the horizon for a dawn that wasn't coming. When I looked back he was there, darker than the gloom and taller, more hulking than he had left, too big now to perch on the bed. I began to fear just how big he might become. "Look," I said. "If we're playing a game I need to know what we're playing for. What if I can't guess and I lose?" He just loitered there to my left, too large for me to get a sense of. "If you lose," he said, a voice now lower and darker, "you lose the game. But the game is why you're here. All of this is the game. You don't want to lose the game, do you?" He was talking about something greater than what met the eye. I thought I was playing for my survival. The 50/50 rule. But how could I know what to say? "Your name is Chemo," I said firmly, as though my confidence alone might make it true. "No!" the ape boomed. "Wrong again." And it turned its back, padding with great meaty hands towards the door. "Once more I will ask you," he added. "One hour." I lay there trembling somewhere near sleep, watching how the night fills the little spaces in everything. I tried to think. The ape will visit four times, four rounds of chemo. He's growing each time. I halted myself awake. This was it, I was officially mad. Laying there in the dark, trying to guess the name of an imaginary ape I had crossed the line marked 'disturbed'. My sheets were soaked so I kicked them down and off and climbed out of bed. I pressed the buzzer for the nurse and stood watching the little window in my door as a bell rang somewhere far off. "Besides," the tougher, more awake part of my brain said aloud, now taking control, "that stupid monkey's name was Cancer." I got out of bed, too afraid to go back to sleep.

Monday June 30 2008. Course 2: Day 22.

I was shivering, my body crying out for something I couldn't give it. Thirsty for something it had no signal for. To cover up was too hot, to uncover too cold. This was the horrible limbo that surfaced sometimes, capricious and cruel. There was no way around it, only through.

Somewhere down the hall the ward hummed with the sounds of another morning, sounds that could have belonged to any office or workplace. I had been removed from the centre of all that life, and was feeling increasingly isolated inside this box. Contact with anyone else was minimal, and I just tended to bounce around like Steve McQueen's baseball in 'The Great Escape,' chasing off the hours until Mary arrived.

I was now desperate to know what my blood counts were doing. It was Day 22 and there was a good chance they would be on their way back up. I had asked to see my counts a couple of times in the past few days, but the nurses had got tangled up in other things and forgotten to print them off. But in the afternoon I collared one of the sisters and asked to see that morning's results. I waited nervously in my room for over half an hour, looking from wall to clock to a fixed point in space and back again, until a folded piece of paper landed on my bed. I raised my eyebrows. It was more than I was expecting. Haemoglobin (or HB): 11.4, neutrophils 0.7, platelets 121 and white cell count 2.0. All were in much better shape than when I had been sent home from Chesterfield. I was on my way out of the tunnel of Chemo 2 and though I could have felt joy, and I did to a certain degree, what I mainly felt was an itch to get home. My urges to get out of that room had just multiplied ten-fold now I knew I was ready. Though the figures were good I suspected they weren't high enough for the doctors to send me packing yet. I sensed one of those "before the end of the week" conversations coming on.

Tuesday July 1 2008. Course 2: Day 23.

I was up most of the night with my stomach doing cartwheels. It was making me fidget, and no position was comfortable. I watched midnight become 1 a.m., and then 2 a.m. become 3. In the end I could stand it no longer and crossed the side hallway to the toilet and jabbed my fingers to the back of my throat until I was happy I'd vomited everything from my stomach. I drank a glass of milk from the nurses' station and walked back to my room, surprised at how many others were awake. I flopped back into bed, surrendering myself to sleep. When it came, I found myself at the edge of a huge golden cornfield. The sun baked the stalks as they gently whispered in the breeze. I stood and listened to the stillness for a while, before stepping forward into the midst of the corn. It was a full foot above my head in height but parted welcomingly as I moved through its orderly rows. I reached out, feeling contrast between the soft heads of the corn and the occasional sharpness of the stalks below. Time wandered on and I paused, unsure of what direction I had come through the repetition of sentries. I listened. There was a far-off bird song carried somewhere overhead, but something else as well. Something quiet but becoming more insistent. It was a bell. The jingle of a small bell being rung by hand. I knew at once to run from it, that whoever or whatever called me with that bell meant to do me harm. And so I ran, leaving behind the track, and ploughing blindly through the heart of the field, its crop no longer yielding to let me pass. The harder I swept aside a stalk as I ran the more firmly anchored it seemed to be to the dry earth. Despite the thrash and breathlessness of my progress I could hear the bell, that bell, all the time getting closer, surprising me by sounding suddenly to my other side, causing me to spin. The bell rang at once right ahead of me, jangling every so softly in the fading light, from what felt like merely feet away, just behind the next few curtains of corn. I saw a shadow move and I was filled with a dread that threatened to fix me there. But I backed and turned, finding in me fight enough to run. I smashed through a row of corn, snapping one over, and I cut off to the side, spotting a corner in the shape of the planting, a meeting of two tracks and what must be a navigation point. I made for it, kicking away from the soft ring of that bell, like a wind chime from some forgotten summer. I pounded for the corner, slowing slightly to take it and was plunged, first one foot then the other, into a bath of mud. I sunk and splashed right up to the waist, caught in the vacuum of the pool. I tried to move a leg but found it bolted. My hips even, were locked into the earth, it was useless. No amount of squirming would have gotten me anything but deeper entrenched. I felt my body start to slide down into the mire and was conscious of the sinking of the sun behind the corn. In seconds my neck and head alone were showing above the dirt. My eyes were caught by something glinting on the floor just feet ahead. It was a tiny bell, standing as if placed, ready to chime its subdued song. The mud was cold as it filled my eyes and I went under.

I woke to find it was dawn, and I lay cocooned in bed watching the colours of a new day bleed into the night. I could find no meaning in my dream. I was ill, tortured. Nothing more could I attach to it, other than my dreams of late seemed united by themes of drowning and fear of the unknown.

I tried to fill up the hours before breakfast by tidying up a bit or reading, but time really can stretch the belief that it is constant. At long last, the doctors got to me at the tail-end of their rounds. It was one of the physicians I had seen only once before but had liked straight away. He tried to be funny a fair bit of the time and for a lot of that he got it right. He told me my counts were looking good and that they should be able to pack me off "before the weekend." It was only Tuesday. I said I hoped for sooner. "Well the thing is," he said, "I tend to err on the side of pessimism when it comes to discharging people so as not to disappoint. But you may be out sooner, who knows? It all depends on your counts really." The benchmark seemed to be a white cell count of 3. Mine was currently 2. He recommended I discuss it again with Dr. Snell on his rounds on Thursday, which was, coincidentally, my target to be out of there. Next I wanted to know about the timing of my two remaining treatments around the wedding. Since it now seemed impossible to get them both done before, we were going to be left with one treatment pre-September and one pretty large gap somewhere. The choice therefore seemed to be, did I leave a few weeks now before starting Course 3 and have a big gap on the other side too, or was only one long gap more advisable. In the end his advice helped more than I think he realised. "First of all, we don't know how much merit there even is in having a fourth course of treatment. We know we need three but it isn't clear how much a fourth course aids in stopping things coming back." That was useful to know straight away, though it conflicted with some things I'd heard to date. "But it's not great to have big gaps between treatments, the theory being it gives the bad cells chance to re-establish themselves." He gripped each end of the stethoscope around his neck and went on. "In some countries they just keep you in hospital the whole time and as soon as you're well enough, they blast you again, we don't do that because most people can't handle it. What I'm getting at though is one longer gap after Course 3 is better than two medium-sized gaps." That was what I wanted to hear, a longer gap for the wedding and no need for too much guilt about it. There was still a worry about leaving long breaks at all. Yes, this was my wedding but did I really want to take risks with my life over it? Would I look back and think "If only I'd got straight on with Course 4." I had one more question, why had I been put on Metronidazole, which I knew to be the antibiotic used to treat C-diff? The doctor smiled and looked at the floor. He didn't seem too sure himself. "Well the good news is that you don't actually have C-diff. The stool samples you've given us have been negative so ..." He looked down at my drug charts. "What I think happened was that Dr. Snell put you on Metronidazole before he had the sample results, as a precaution." I paused. "And now?" He seemed cheery all of a sudden. "Well it's not doing you any harm, it's just that it's not doing you any direct good, I suppose. It's not a bad thing to be on, the drug that wards off C-diff – you are in hospital after all."

Wednesday July 2 2008. Course 2: Day 24.

I woke up, around 4 a.m., drenched. For the fourth night in a row I had to buzz for some fresh sheets. Mary had told me the night sweats were something to do with my body purging all the stuff it didn't need as it regenerated. I didn't know if that was true or not but it sounded plausible. All I knew was that it was getting embarrassing asking for the sheets, I didn't want a reputation as a bed-wetter, though that's exactly what I was in some sense. I was feeling stronger. I could feel the infection was behind me and my counts were bouncing back. This was the home straight. I was through it. Had it been easier than Course 1, as doctors had promised? Easier, yes; easy, no. I had come in this time with healthy counts, rather than those of someone in the grip of an acute disease. But I'd still passed through a couple of the lower regions to get to the other side. The bite of an infection when you have no immune system is something difficult to describe in its awfulness. Once it starts, you know you are guaranteed to feel wretched for at least a week. I had escaped with only one infection this time, something I put, in part, down to my vigilance. But I had dodged most of the factors which made Course 1 so hellish. Sleep, blessed sleep. I had slept and the difference that made to my mental health couldn't be overstated. My mental demons had been born and fed during sleepless nights and, though I had still heard from them lately, their influence was much more restricted. Then there was my mouth which had mercifully, miraculously stayed free of the lesions and ulcers I had suffered before. They had stopped me eating and even smiling, so to be free of them was a huge benefit. I had also kept most of my weight on. I had lost only a few pounds all in all, a stark contrast to last time when I lost a stone-and-a-half, leaving me so weak I could hardly walk. I was looking forward to coming out in much better shape than I had last time, when I was practically an invalid for the first week.

As I looked out over Sheffield, longing to get out there, as a free man again, Tara, one of the ward sisters, called in to ask if I was free of the diarrhoea. What I told her wasn't a lie as such, for the most part I was free of it, other than the occasional episode. My thinking was that I didn't want anything to get in the way of my being sent home so I wanted them all to be happy I was tip-top all round. Tara told me; in that case, they would be moving me back onto the ward. I allowed myself the smallest laugh. This would be my fourth bed on the same ward in the space of two weeks. They could have moved me to the roof as far as I was concerned, I was going home soon.

When I had lugged my considerable hulk of stuff down the hall to my new bed, I found I was to be next to an old friend. Simon, aka Grumpy, and I would be bunking up once again. I couldn't tell at what stage of his cycle Simon was at right away, though I gathered his counts were on the way down. Essentially he was at the counterpoint to where I was. He seemed convinced that he had an infection already and may have been right, knowing his luck. He made sure everybody was aware that he was ill and felt shivery. Good luck to him, but I was busy projecting a front of good health. I was concentrating on exuding wellness so that everybody, staff mostly, would pick up on it and decide that this boy was taking up a bed and would be better out from under everyone's feet.

It seemed to work straight away, such was the mastery of my performance. The doctor I had seen the day before reached me on his rounds and told me I could go home, pretty much whenever I wanted. I was a bit taken aback by the suddenness of it, but doctors seemed to prefer things that way. "Now you might choose to hang around until tomorrow morning to see Dr. Snell and he can answer any questions you have about things from here on in." Although it meant killing another day, that sounded sensible and I said so. He nodded, "The other thing is a bone marrow biopsy, which we could even arrange for tomorrow as well." I instinctively agreed, realising later I was consenting to an entirely optional procedure which I hated. Dr. Cowdrey had explained to me weeks earlier that they did not routinely do bone marrow biopsies after Course 2, as the next action was always the same i.e. proceed with Course 3. This rendered the result academic, why put the patient through the discomfort of it? But part of me wanted to know, wanted to hear that word 'remission'. Even Dr. Cowdrey would have been curious to see the result; I was sure, despite what he'd said.

As I pondered the prospect of another bone marrow Austin, one of the nursing staff, dropped on my bed the results of that morning's blood tests. I picked them up and did a double-take, saying the word, "Jesus" too loud so that everybody looked up. Everything had shot right up, some by around half, others had nearly doubled. Jesus indeed. I had smashed right through the threshold for being sent home. Mary was over the moon. She desperately wanted me at home and was finding it increasingly hard to cope with things as they were.

Earlier that day she had met with an Occupational Health Adviser through work and filled out a couple of tests which had scored her as 18 out of 21 for depression and 20 out of 21 for anxiety. As fantastic as our friends and family were, the initial shock of my diagnosis had passed and the dust had settled. People were going back to their lives. Of course they were. I would not want or expect anyone to put anything off on my account. In fact hearing they had done so would upset me. But there was no life for Mary to go back to; in some ways we had brought that on ourselves. The first course had been so intense we had asked people to back off a little and give Mary and me some space. I think they took it to heart and some went to the other extreme.

Now that I knew I was getting out, the necessary veil of optimism about my surroundings dropped, and I could see the ward for what it was, a grave and oppressive place. People around me shook and shivered and vomited in cardboard trays. They slept, gaunt and open-mouthed, as though the very life was being drawn from them in their comas. The staff were wonderful but what were they really doing? What could they hope to do but stem the constant ebb of life from everyone. It is an irreconcilably sad place despite the air of hope, and the only way we can live there and not go mad is by becoming numb to it, distant, as though not really there at all. Now, and only now, did I allow myself to inhabit Ground Zero for a while. I'd soon had my fill and flipped the switch again to turn out the lights.

Thursday July 3 2008. Course 2: Day 25.

When I opened my eyes at 5 a.m. I knew I would not be getting back to sleep. My stomach was a nervous knot of energy. I began quietly tidying my things as the occasional night-shift nurse paced past in the dimly-lit corridor. I checked again my list of questions for Dr. Snell. I hadn't attempted to commit them to memory in case I forgot any of them, though they were only a handful in number. People around me were stirring. I gathered that everyone in the bay was having, or had, undergone chemo so quite why I assumed them to be sleeping I didn't know. But daylight was slowly filling the room through the window's breach in the wall, and with it everyone became less concerned with muffling their movements. The volume switch was slowly being turned and the hospital was gently shaking everyone awake.

I watched the clock tick over in the corner of the breakfast news, telling myself I would wait until certain times of the morning before beginning different tasks that made up getting ready. Ward rounds tended to take place later on a Thursday, so I knew I had an extra hour or so to kill. I absent-mindedly chewed my breakfast, hoping it would be my last meal in the place. Shortly afterwards I managed to dive into one of the bathrooms with a shower, no mean feat, as several of the other doors bore signs reserving them for certain bays as part of infection control procedures to stamp out the diarrhoea bug. I selfishly took as long as I could getting ready, desperate for some of the long minutes to wash away with the water.

Three chapters and half a dozen Sudoku puzzles later, the doctors assembled around my bed.

Dr. Snell and I exchanged something of a 'job well done' smile. "Here we are," he said, before asking where I intended to have my next course of treatment. This was something Mary and I had agonised over. The Hallamshire had a bigger wallet that was obvious in everything they did. It was better staffed in that there were more bodies on shift, there was always a doctor or five around the place, even at night. They thought nothing of sending patients for scans, tests or X-rays, or giving them some expensive new drug that other NHS Trusts probably couldn't legislate for. Even the food was better. But I felt drawn back to the Royal at Chesterfield, partly, and perhaps foolishly, through loyalty. I greatly respected the two consultants there and knew that, together with Alison, the ward sister, they felt terrible about me having to go to Sheffield at all. I felt their commitment to getting me well went deeper than it simply being their job. Though the same could be said of Dr. Snell and co. at the Hallamshire in all fairness. What swung it, as with so many things in life, was money. Cold, hard cash. We could ill-afford the expense of Mary driving to Sheffield and back each day and parking while there. The hospitals were about on a par so it would be something as trivial as money that would decide it. I felt as though I was doing someone a disservice by this being the case. Perhaps it was Dr. Snell. Perhaps it was myself. Either way, I felt dirty and treacherous by answering "Chesterfield". "Okay, fine," Dr. Snell replied without a hint of bitterness or disappointment.

The one last thing I needed from him was honesty about my aspirations for my wedding. How was I best to proceed from here? It was still possible, in theory, to cram in the two remaining treatments before September 12 and be recovered, but it was reliant on a dizzying number of variables, not least my own ability to bounce back quickly. It looked more likely that we would have to opt for one course before and one after, but this left a break in between of around a month, something we thought wouldn't be advisable. Dr. Snell listened to me stating my case and, as he rubbed his hands together in front of him, I sensed this was somehow a conversation he was uncomfortable with. In the wedding we had an obstacle which couldn't just be pushed aside without emotional consequences. It had to be negotiated sensitively but, ultimately, involved a decision only I could make. Dr. Snell paused thoughtfully. "When did you book your wedding?" he asked. "Before all this started." He nodded. "Well, it may be that you decide to put the date back to take some of the pressure off yourselves." His voice suddenly sped up. "But I'm not saying that's what you should do or would have to do." Something drooped inside of me. He clearly thought the date was ill-placed but didn't want to be the one to say it outright. It would have been so much easier if he had. For some reason I felt uneasy, cornered. "Look," I said, "the pressure isn't what worries me. I just need to know how bad it would be to leave that four-week gap between courses. I know it's probably inadvisable but I need to know just how inadvisable it would be." Dr. Snell nodded again, rubbed his hands. "Okay. In some other countries they don't leave much gap at all, may be a day or so after the counts start to pick up." I recognised this story, having been told it by another doctor days earlier. "We don't do that here because, psychologically, most people simply wouldn't be able to take it. But, medically speaking, it's probably the most effective way to treat the disease because the bad cells don't have as much time to grow back. Do you understand?" I did. There was a clear message. Pitching treatments either side of the wedding would be a massive gamble.

If we allowed such a gap and the cancer returned further down the line, we would forever curse ourselves for pressing ahead. Part of me had always known the best option for my health was to put the wedding back, particularly as we also had to factor in a stem cell harvest somewhere between the final two courses. But I had always dismissed this voice, believing everything would fit in somehow even though the numbers didn't stack up. I wondered how I would raise the issue with Mary. She would support me if I decided the date should move, but in the short term she would be devastated. People on the outside looking in would say it was just a date, something which could be changed. But to us it had been more than that, a point in time we had both looked forward to for 18 months and, with recent developments, had become a target for my recovery. It was to be the full-stop after all of this and the biggest party of our lives. To move the date, personally, would feel like a further concession to the disease, which I saw as my opponent. I had set myself that target and I was far too competitive to relinquish it unless I really had to. There was also the fact that the date itself was now a matter of weeks away. Invitations had been sent, replies received. Photographers, videographers, chauffeur, hairdressers had been booked, there was no guarantee they could or would just agree on a new date. Who, of our friends and family, might not be able to attend on some other day at such short notice? When put back to? Part of me was angry at my doctors at Chesterfield, who had assured us they could get me well for the wedding date and there would be no need to move it. But things change, I knew. The unexpected happens. They believed that at the time and so did we. That belief was fading fast.

I watched Dr. Snell and his colleagues move on to the next patient in the bay, another poor soul at some other point in the same ghastly timeline I was riding. He had only his treatment to focus on. Whether this made things easier or not I would never know. All I could think was, despite all the complications, the wedding offered me comfort and hope, something to strive for. Despite everything this seemed like the perfect time in our lives to be getting married rather than the worst possible time, as some may have believed.

I spotted Andrea, the Hallamshire's Transplant Coordinator, in the hallway and I asked for a quick word. We made our way to an empty room on the ward and settled into a big green armchair each. Andrea came across as an extremely bubbly character, who would drop a big beaming smile into the middle of a sentence without warning. This personality came out, despite the seriousness of her work and I for one found it comforting, if a bit disconcerting.

I was keen to know more about the timing of the stem cell harvesting procedure, and if it was an avenue that would still be pursued if I reverted back to Chesterfield for my next treatment. Andrea assured me that it was. The procedure itself would be factored in some time after I had recovered from the third course at a time that could be agreed with everybody. That told me little I didn't already know. "The harvest itself will be done one of two ways," Andrea went on. "Either via the machine that skims off the stem cells from the blood or, more likely, direct from the bone marrow under general anaesthetic." I raised my eyebrows. This was news to me. Andrea herself had left me a leaflet weeks earlier which documented only the harvest via a machine, I imagined was similar to dialysis. Now I was being told I was "more likely" to be put to sleep for a harvest direct from my bone marrow. "If it was done that way," Andrea said, "it usually means a two-night stay in hospital. Your red cell count would go down a little, but most people are well enough to go home again the next day." The longer we talked about the stem cell harvest, the more I realised that, should I ever need them back, I was in trouble. They would only be re-introduced should I have first undergone a transplant of someone else's stem cells which had failed to 'take' in my bone marrow. It sounded as though, before undergoing a transplant, a patient was 'prepped' with high doses of chemo and radiotherapy, something which terrified me. I was still holding on to the hope of walking away from all of this with my fertility. If it was to come to a transplant that would almost certainly be lost. Yes, I had a sample on ice in Sheffield, but I dearly wanted to do things naturally and felt sure Mary thought the same, though she hadn't yet said so. If anything, this process had shown us what little time any of us truly have, and perhaps trying to have a family should be something we should go for sooner rather than later. We had talked about it and had agreed that much. Mary had told me that, even if I didn't make it, she would want that part of me to live on. That was what I hoped she might feel, though I would have fully understood if not. I said to Andrea that we were now leaning towards the idea of having one treatment before the wedding and one afterwards, as trying to cram them both in beforehand seemed a stretch. "Oh, yes," she said. "You'd have to be superhuman." Something cracked inside of me. What she had just said sounded, to me in my stupidly competitive brain, like a challenge.

She thought two courses before the wedding wasn't possible. A part of me still thought it was, and was itching to go for it, to get them both out of the way and not have to move the wedding at all. It would be a massive gamble to take it on. I risked being a wreck on my wedding day, something I would always regret. But whatever we decided would have its inherent risks and down-sides. I didn't know I would be able to handle two quick-fire rounds of chemo, with drugs I had no idea how I'd react to. I could get a string of infections or take an age to recover my blood counts. I might go the whole hog and actually go mad this time. That would certainly make for an interesting wedding speech. I needed to speak with Mary about it all first. I knew she would say it was down to me and she would support me in whatever I chose, but I felt it should be a joint decision. Maybe I just knew it was going to be the hardest decision of my life and I didn't want to make it alone.

I said goodbye for now to Andrea, feeling, not for the first time, a little lost in it all. It seemed that no-one could offer me the guarantees on dates that I needed. That was the nature of battling leukaemia there were no guarantees at all. Nobody could say anything for sure. Just before we left the room, I asked a question which had just popped into my head: what percentage of leukaemia patients go on to need a transplant? Andrea nodded and flashed a smile, though this time it looked forced, troubled. "That's a very good question," she began, "and one which you are well within your rights to ask." She paused, before talking around the subject for a full minute or two. But she had ducked the question completely. Perhaps I wouldn't like the answer and it would serve me no good to know. The fact that she didn't tell me was answer enough.

We went our separate ways out of the room and I walked around to the lift area to meet Mary, who had texted me minutes earlier to say she had arrived. She was full of beans, excited about taking me home. I tried to share in that but my thoughts had already bounded onwards to my next course and beyond. Mary picked up on the flatness in my voice, seeing right through me as she always did. It was clear to her that whatever Dr. Snell had said had knocked me back. I told her everything as we sat there watching the irregular pulse of staff and visitors flowing in and out of the lifts. I told her what Dr. Snell had said, what he hadn't said and what he hadn't needed to say. I could see the tears in her eyes before I'd even finished talking. "We're going to have to cancel the wedding, aren't we?" "No," I returned. "We won't have to cancel anything." I didn't know if that was true. A non-vocal half of me thought not. "We can work round the date we have. One way or another we're keeping it." I had to reign myself in, realising I was making promises which were built on forever shifting sands.

We collected my things from my bedside and I said farewell to the others in the bay. There was a certain unspoken camaraderie there, though I'd known them all only a matter of days, such that we could all wish each other good luck and mean it with a depth most people couldn't understand. I said goodbye to the nursing team, slightly disappointed that none of those who had helped bounce me back when I was low were on shift. We left deflated, both of us thinking too far ahead to really enjoy this time together on the outside.

Friday – Monday: July 4 – 7 2008. Course 2: Days 26 - 29.

Being home again this time was a different experience. I was in much better health from the off, so wasn't so limited in what I was able to do. It was fair to say I was appreciating the break less than I had the first time. My time in hospital had been far less traumatic and, in a perverse way, I couldn't wait to get back in and start the next course. At least then I was on the treadmill and getting somewhere, rather than the prospect hanging somewhere in my line of sight the whole time. We meandered from place to place, both of us distant. Mary kept telling me I looked like I was on another planet some of the time, but she was elsewhere too. I recognised the building in her emotions and knew that at some point they would boil over in a big way. There was nothing I could do to diffuse that situation, I knew, just be there to listen and pick up the pieces if I could.

We sat down one afternoon for a meal in a pub's beer garden and couldn't help but overhear a woman talking about shoes and handbags for a full hour. How blissfully ignorant she was, we both agreed, to be driven by such things. We talked about the wedding every couple of hours, and how we should try and place treatments around it. But we often ended up talking ourselves into despondency, while arriving at no decisions. The problem was that our date was so awkwardly placed it gave every option its drawbacks. My two remaining courses of treatment could be squeezed in before the day and I could be mostly recovered but it relied on an awful lot of luck. If the ward was closed again or I recovered slowly it would derail the whole plan. To pitch the courses either side of the wedding would mean a four or five week break between treatments which felt like a risk. It would also mean me going back into hospital on the Monday after the wedding, hardly what either of us wanted. If we had to put the date back we would both be devastated. It was something we had looked forward to so much. It had been our target and our anchor through all of this, to lose it now would be really hard to take. Plus, when would we put it back to? We risked moving the date into the path of any further treatment, if and when that was deemed necessary. If our date had been just a few days either side of where it was, the decision would have made itself. As it was, we were going to have to call it.

Though Mary and I were both on the same side, the decision was pulling us apart. We kept arguing over unrelated things, often when Mary would vent her frustration at people who didn't deserve it. I spoke up on one occasion and she stormed out of the house with the car keys, telling me she hoped she would crash so she didn't have to think about any of this anymore. I sat in a heap by the door waiting for her to return, watching the distorted shapes of people and cars moving past the frosted glass. I was relieved when I finally saw her car draw up against the pavement. Mary breezed in past me and went to the fridge, pouring herself some alcoholic mixer and went upstairs. I sat there on the living room floor for a minute or two, trying to find the words to say, if they existed. There really were no assurances I could give about any of it. It still seemed so unreal but this was happening to us. This was what was left of our lives and we had to find a way to move on and be happy again.

I rose to my feet and climbed the stairs. I found Mary sitting on our bed, flicking through a wedding magazine. Her drink was half gone already, her face spilling over with tears. I sat beside her and took the magazine and drink from her hands. She resisted and turned her head away, showing me she had already put a barrier up against whatever I had found to say. I looked at her for a moment longer, feeling the grief emanating from her every movement. "You look so angry," was what I chose as an opener, though I wasn't sure why. "I am angry, Richard. I'm angry at you, I'm angry at me, I'm angry at God and I'm angry at everyone we know." If there was any kind of reply to that I sure as hell didn't know what it was. I reached out to touch her but she pulled away. "No" she snapped. "We should just call the wedding off. I don't love you anymore." That felt like a punch in the stomach. I searched for eye contact but couldn't pin her gaze down. Wounded, I stood and made for the door, turning to see if I could catch her eye but she was fixed on something out of the window. I floated down the stairs in a daze. I intended to leave the house. To get in the car or just start walking. We both needed some time apart to think. But when I got to the door I had no energy to go any further, and found myself collapsed on the floor once again. I would understand if that was how she felt.

I didn't want to see her tied to me if I was going to fade away. I wanted more than anything in the world for her to be happy, whatever that meant for me. I heard Mary coming down the stairs and she soon appeared in the doorway, crying harder than ever. She dropped to her knees beside me and took my arm. "I do love you," she pleaded."I love you too much. I wish I didn't love you so much and then this wouldn't be so hard." Her soul was so tortured she could hardly speak. It cut me up to see her this way. I had never asked for any of this. People told me it wasn't my fault, and often I believed them. But this awful thing was channelling itself through me and hurting everyone I cared about. For that much, I was truly sorry. "I'm terrified, Richard," Mary managed between gasped breaths. "I'm terrified you're not going to get better and you're going to leave me here by myself." I got a true sense of the weight of her pain for the first time. I held her as tightly as I could.

Tuesday July 8 2008. Course 2: Day 30.

We had arranged to go into the hospital at Chesterfield and talk with Alison about fitting treatments around the wedding date. As soon as I stepped inside the building I was hit by that smell of disinfectant that had provided the backdrop to my descent into the abyss the last time I was here. I held Mary's hand a little tighter. We followed the maze of corridors to Cavendish Suite and I announced myself at the desk. The receptionist seemed to know who I was already and told us to take a seat while she went to find Alison.

Within minutes she had appeared, smiley as ever, and summoned us to a private room at the end of the hall. It seemed we had both brought an array of papers with us. Hers documented the next two courses of chemotherapy. I would be randomised to one of six courses of treatment. Four of them trialled different doses of Cytarabine, the drug I had been given on my first two courses and either with or without a drug called Mylotarg. Now we were into my third and fourth courses, known as consolidation chemotherapy, the approach was slightly different. We knew I was in remission after Course 1, so now the number of leukaemic cells in my body should be minimal. If Courses 1 and 2 were airstrikes, 3 and 4 were much more targeted attacks on what was left. Mylotarg seemed to be about as targeted as the experts knew how to be. The drug carries another chemotherapy agent, Ozogamicin, directly to cancerous cells, ones showing the CD33 protein, and locks onto them. It was thought the drug may not affect normal cells within the body. None of the above could be said with complete certainty Mylotarg was yet to be approved for use outside of clinical trials in the UK. Then there were two other possible courses of treatment, ones I wished to avoid: the affectionately titled MACE, administered either with or without Mylotarg. MACE was a loose acronym of the drugs which comprised the treatment: Amsacrine, Cytarabine and Etoposide. What put me off this treatment, aside from the fact it was two new drugs for my body to contend with, was the necessity to be attached to a drip continuously 24 hours a day for 5 days.

I felt sure I would be drawn for this programme, for no other reason than my aversion to it. Chain yourself to a beeping, whirring pole with dickey wheels for an hour of two and you'll begin to get an idea of how restrictive it is. If I'd had a choice, which of course I didn't, I would have gone for one of the Cytarabine courses with Mylotarg. Though the drug was not yet fully proven, it sounded like a step in the right direction. But the nature of the trials was such that half would receive it, half would not.

I took comfort in what Dr. Strong had told me at the beginning that the trials had been running long enough for them to have known by now if any treatment was significantly better than the others. Before I could be randomised for any of the courses, I first needed to sign a consent form. I never thought, in this life or the next, I would so eagerly sign up for medical experiments.

With the formalities out of the way, we moved on to the hard part. We just needed to know, needed someone to tell us, if we should put back the wedding. We mapped out the timescale once more, something the pair of us was sick of doing by now, while Alison listened in thoughtfully, and we asked what risks were attached to delaying the fourth course of treatment. "Well, I've spoken to both Drs. Strong and Cowdrey ahead of meeting you today," Alison began. "And the simple answer is that we don't know." I sighed, somehow always knowing that would be the advice. "Nobody really leaves a gap like that, unless their counts are slow to recover. People get on the programme of treatment and undergo the treatments one after the other, so we don't know what difference the delay would make. Dr. Strong has offered to email the trial's professors to ask their opinion. If anybody would know it would be them." I looked at Mary and could tell she wanted to cry. "I just feel a bit let down by it all," Mary said. "The doctors told us at the start that we didn't need to cancel anything. Now we're much further down the line and nobody knows what to say." She shrugged. "We just don't know what to do." Alison nodded. She understood, I felt sure, but we were no closer to making a decision. "There is the option to get both treatments in before," Alison said. "You were talking about coming back into hospital on Monday, but what if we could do sooner than that maybe Thursday or Friday of this week. We have a patient, in your old room, as it happens, who we're hoping will be well enough to discharge at the end of this week. If we could get you in then, if you wanted to and assuming your bloods were okay, that could buy you a few more days." My first thoughts were positive, it felt like progress, but it was tinged with fear and regret about going back in. But this was surely an opportunity we couldn't pass up. Mary was nodding at me. "Okay," I said. "That would keep our options open, thank you." If I was back in by Friday it would mean I had had just over a week on the outside.

Considering I had left Sheffield early, that is to say before Day 28 of the cycle, it could be said we had won back some time. Every day was truly precious to us now if I was to stand at the end of the aisle rather than sit in a wheelchair. Assuming I could get into hospital that week, the chance of getting both treatments in pre-wedding would be bolstered, though it still seemed very ambitious. That much we knew, but there was no easy way out of where we found ourselves.

Wednesday July 9 2008. Course 2: Day 31.

Knowing my time now looked limited on the outside, we got to work with what I needed to be present for as far as planning the wedding was concerned. We went to get me fitted for my suit and arranged an appointment to give the details for the marriage licence. I was also busy trying to put some weight back on, having lost more than I thought, about 8 lbs. in all, while I was in hospital in Sheffield. My weight had continued to come down for a couple of days after being discharged as I got rid of all the extra fluid I was carrying. But I was without the ravenous hunger which had driven me to bulk back up last time. I knew that, with two rapid-fire rounds of chemo ahead, I risked dropping a fair bit of weight and looking skeletal on our wedding photos. I knew I had to be proactive with supplements to keep that loss to a minimum. Weight loss would also mean a loss of strength and stamina on the day, which would impact on my ability to enjoy it; even with the adrenaline boosts I hoped my body would grant me. But for now I was feeling pretty healthy in myself and had my fingers crossed for a storming result on the blood test Alison had taken from me days earlier. If my counts were sluggish it could delay my treatment or point to some kind of problem. Despite feeling well and being able to function more or less normally, I was conscious that others were being very protective of me. I got a seat first; I got fed first, and was constantly asked if I was okay. No amount of protestation from me would have put an end to it, friends and family were being exactly that, and I was willing to put up with the awkwardness of it to let them feel they were helping in some small way.

In the evening we attended Marion's choir concert, and, afterwards, she practically begged me to stop stacking away the chairs. Several members of the choir, who had very kindly volunteered to sing at the wedding, greeted me with hugs and words of encouragement which was very heart-warming. Some people found it hard to say anything reassuring to me. They were no expert, they probably thought, how could they offer me hollow messages of hope. All I knew was that any expression of belief added to my own. There are no entry qualifications for faith.

Thursday July 10 2008. Course 2: Day 32.

"Did I wake you?" Alison asked. I pressed the phone to my ear and blinked at the clock. "No," I lied. It was 9 a.m. on Thursday. "It sounds like I did," she laughed. This was the phone call we had been waiting for. I sat up. "No, no. I'm awake. Any news?" "Yes. We have a bed for you today. It isn't the one I was expecting but we have one. If you are able to come in this morning you could see the doctors and we can get your drugs ordered from pharmacy. Then you could come back tomorrow to begin your treatment." I was nodding. This was what I had hoped for. "Yes please," I said. "That sounds ideal. Thank you." For the first time we were gaining time instead of losing it. Each day could make the difference on the other side. We got together a minimum of my things and headed in.

Manning the desk on Durrant Ward was a familiar face; Wayne, who had accompanied me on my sperm sample expedition to Sheffield months earlier. It was nice to see him, and a few of the others I knew who were busy dashing around, short staffed as always. I had seen the other side to that coin at the Hallamshire. But I had great respect and admiration for the job they did. I knew that Wayne himself had gone into nursing later in life after spending several months in hospital in a wheelchair. He must have been inspired, just as I was, by the everyday people doing extraordinary things for others. It compelled you to want to join them; made whatever you were doing before seem trivial and vacuous. I didn't feel I had what it took to do their job, however, not at this stage of my life at least. Wayne pointed to the nearest side room, the one I had been originally admitted to before being moved down the hall. We filed in and took a seat. I looked around and realised I had an uncanny memory for the place, being as I was able to recall every undulation in the wall, every mark or imperfection on the surfaces around me.

We were soon joined by Drs. Strong, Cowdrey and Woodward, as well as Alison and the planning for Course 3 could begin. They asked me about my experiences at Sheffield, and I passed on that the doctors there thought the drug that had spawned that awful rash was most likely Tazocin one of the antibiotics used as treatment for infections. They flicked through my notes and saw that I had indeed been given that during my first course, so it was added as one to avoid. "How were my blood results?"I asked, suddenly remembering. Dr. Cowdrey nodded, "Your counts were excellent," he said, stressing the last word. I swallowed, relieved. Anything else would have been a worry. "And which drugs have I been randomised to this time?" There was a pause in the room, and instantly I knew the answer. "Erm, yes," Alison began. "I'm afraid it's the ones you didn't want. You've been randomised to MACE."

Course 3

Friday – Wednesday: July 11 – 16 2008. Course 3: Days 1 – 5: Chemo Days 1 - 5.

It was soon apparent just how much of a pain MACE was to administer, let alone receive. First, I was hooked up to a glucose solution drip, as the first drug, Amsacrine, ran through with that rather than saline. After the Amsacrine had gone through for an hour, it was washed through with glucose, then the line was flushed with normal saline. Next we had Etoposide for one hour, followed by another saline rinse, before the main event, 500ml of Cytarabine solution, could be hooked up to go in at a crawl over the course of 20 hours. I seemed to be forever pressing my buzzer to tell the nurses that one bag or the other had finished and I was ready for the next one.

The effects were noticeable before too long. Amsacrine gave my urine a bright yellow tinge. All of them gave me nausea. It seemed to be the Cytarabine, however, which made me feel the most nauseated, despite the snail-pace of its delivery. I sank back into the familiar rhythms of rejecting food, of food repulsing me. I seemed to vomit whether I ate or not. Often I could picture something I'd be happy to have a crack at eating, but these changed from one delicacy to another with the wind, and none of them were on the menu at this diner. I'd find myself staring at the food choices for too long, scanning for something, anything that might fire a pang of hunger. But it was little use. However, I did manage to keep down a good few shots of Calogen, a milky strawberry drink which packed a 400 calorie kick in each serving, as the days progressed – something I prayed would keep some meat on my bones.

As the days ticked by I began vomiting more and more, I had foolishly thought my constitution might have built up some form of tolerance to these paint-stripper drugs by now; but clearly it had not. My stomach felt as though it was full of battery acid that was burning my insides. The vomiting was just a way of getting that out and I usually felt better afterwards. Course 3 was only a five-day course of drugs and I had my eyes fixed on the end of that when, I hoped, the doctors would let me go home for a few days as my counts began to fall. But I was warned about this sickness, which was different to what I'd had before. And I knew there was a chance my time on the outside this time might not be so blissful because of it, if it persisted.

Thursday July 17 2008. Course 3: Day 6: Chemo Day 6.

Because the MACE drugs took so long to go in, it was actually Day 6 before they were finished. My things were packed long before. I'd spent much of the previous night awake being sick, and listening to some of the ward's lost souls. One man was howling, and not, I suspected, through pain. He would break off to occasionally shout, "You bitch!" After a couple of hours he got bored and went to sleep.

I'd given a blood sample earlier which would tell the doctors how much my counts had come down already and plot a rough trajectory for when they wanted to see me again, but I faced a long wait for the drugs to run through before they could hook me off them. Eventually being free, after five days, felt strange. Dr. Cowdrey called in and said my counts were still high. Mary and I were keen to press for a readmission after the weekend, as this would allow us to attend my step-brother, Ben's wedding, which I'd previously had to begrudgingly rule myself out of. I wasn't sure I would be on top form if I made it along but hoped I'd be okay. I just had a feeling Dr. Cowdrey was going to invite me back in before then. "I think," Dr. Cowdrey said, "we will ask you to come in for clinic on Monday and see what your counts are doing, but it may be the end of next week before we have to get you back." Mary and I shot a smile at each other, that was more than either of us could have been expecting. To have such a long break in the middle would give us both a psychological boost for carrying on. My fear was just how healthy I was likely to be. I could feel MACE had taken a real toll on me and I questioned why one so harsh was still used. For effectiveness, I resolved, could be the only answer.

We gathered my things and prescriptions and made our now famous wheelchair dash for freedom. My things contained, rather sensibly as it turned out, a stock of sick bowls. My time out was to be much more eventful than a similar period during my second course at Sheffield would have been, had I been allowed one. I'd felt strong then, confident. Now my smiles at emancipation masked fears of being pretty unwell.

Friday July 18 2008. Course 3: Day 7.

Ben had contacted me to confirm I would now be coming to his big day tomorrow. I answered confidently that I could, if the invitation still stood. He sounded understandably stressed but was happy to re-jig things to fit me in. He would have been within his rights to advise me to give it a miss. After all, if I collapsed or spent the whole day shivering on a sofa it was not going to please anybody. It was going to be a long day, and I would need to take it slowly. My plan was to spend most of it sitting down smiling sweetly until we were picked up at 12.30. We had a group taxi booked for my dad and Marion, Emma and Dave, and Mary and I. If I started to struggle we would simply have to ring another taxi earlier in the night and skulk off. I felt determined I could make the course but didn't know how much energy I would have for the next day. I was already struggling that day as we went into town to quickly pick me up something to wear to fit the black and white dress code. In between pulling on shirts I felt pretty tired, but imagined tomorrow should see me one day better rather than one day worse.

I was trying to load up on fatty foods during the day once again to compensate, but felt the chemo seemed to have played havoc with my digestion system. I had a horrible fight with heartburn which felt like stones in my chest, and would often cause me to pull up in pain. My stomach felt clogged and heavy with acidic bile, never far from threatening to spill its contents. My guts too were complaining constantly. I was having to tailor what and when I ate for the best. Perhaps the wedding was going to be a stretch. Emma and Dave came up to stay with us that night. I went to bed early.

Saturday July 19 2008. Course 3: Day 8.

The girls took their time curling their hair and generally eking out getting ready over the whole morning, while Dave and I lounged on the sofa. I wasn't too strong on my feet for long, so that suited me fine. When time ran out I pulled on the outfit I'd cobbled together at the last minute, feeling not at all comfortable in it or my own skin. Our taxi turned up early and we piled in, with me crammed next to my dad. I wasn't feeling too talkative which I knew was a bad sign for the day. The drive to Sheffield was slow through back boroughs I didn't know, to an imposing and pretty Masonic Lodge hidden away down a back street. Near to, of all things, Hallamshire Hospital. We seemed hopelessly early, something which invariably happened when we were left to my dad's time-keeping.

We spotted Ben, the glowing groom, straight away in the car park. He had arrived by sports car as a wedding day surprise. What was our excuse? We snuck off to have a little look around the place, plotting where we were going for ceremony, meal, bar etc. People had begun assembling outside and when we came back we started to get pulled into photographs of various permutations. I took a few breaks to sit on the edge of the grass, which was dry and spongy in the sunlight. Mary kept apologising for asking me if I was okay all the time but I wasn't hostile to it in the least. I was feeling pretty interchangeable from one moment to the next, and her constant reassurance was helping prop me up.

Soon it was time for more photos in a beautiful entrance stairwell which spiralled up to the hall in which Ben and his bride-to-be, Jenny, would say their vows. We took our seats beside the aisle while awaiting the entrance of the bride. She looked wonderful in her ivory dress when she finally topped the stairs, and both the happy couple couldn't help but shed a tear as they held hands at last. After a relatively brief ceremony, they said "I do" and I was filled with all the wonder, anticipation, hope, dread and fear I'd been bottling up about our wedding. Our day could never now be what it would have been. It was a case of whether it would now be so much more or less than that. Mary asked if I was thinking about our day. I said I was and she squeezed my hand. I looked at the floor, terrified the whole thing might go horribly sideways.

Downstairs again I settled into an armchair while others stood high above me talking. I was starting to get that sinking feeling in health and was a bit scared by it. I didn't want to cause a scene, and it was time for the meal and speeches. Waiters were buzzing around keenly before we'd even taken our seats and the food, which was excellent I thought, was served up with no delay. I tried to pace myself, knowing there was a better than good chance of seeing my meal again before the night was through. In fact, between the main course and dessert Mary spotted me retching and suggested we go out for five minutes fresh air. I agreed, trying not to meet anyone's gaze on the way out. We settled quietly on a bench by the door for a few minutes while I tried to compose myself.

They had picked a nice day for the wedding, warm and clear. I looked up and saw the winds effortlessly toss the trees, making them lean from one way to the other, and considered what mighty forces were at work around us making nothing but microbes of us and everything we cared about. I felt so powerless. I cuddled into the warmth of Mary beside me, so effortlessly understanding, and felt glad I was not alone. Maybe this would be all the time we had, and if so, I was beyond all gratitude for it. I started to cry, for one reason or another, and we talked for a little longer about the future and things which would have seemed pretty heavy topics to us not long ago. Maybe we were coming over all serious in our old age.

We had to soon move back inside to our seats for the dessert but it took me some time to compose myself and stop looking like I'd actually crept round the back to help the caterers chop onions. Soon after eating, as I'd feared would happen, I was sick a small amount in the toilets. My chest was tight across and heavy, I felt heavily nauseous and I was again struck with diarrhoea. This should have been the first signal of the end to me, but I wanted to stay. For everyone else's sake and to prove some enormous lie I was telling myself. My head spun as I went to exit the toilet and walked straight into the groom himself, Marion's son from her former marriage. He shook my hand warmly, "It's brilliant you could come mate. How are you feeling?" I yanked a series of pulleys and raised a smile, "I wouldn't have missed it. How's the day been and everything.... so far?" "Great. Weird though. Still feels weird. Seems to be going too fast." I wobbled. "Oh? Well." "Listen, when you need to get off just go – its fine." "Cheers, but I'm okay. Don't be worrying about me. Congratulations again."

The next part of the night saw me decamping from our seats in the corner of the bar, where I supped water, to the toilets and back again. People were starting to suggest, more and more, forcefully, that I should be making tracks and Mary was getting beside herself with worry that I was pleading the opposite. I missed the first dance, a choreographed Tango, while I was hurling in the gents, hearing only a distant applause.

Mary had already got together some taxi numbers but I suggested we sit in the main hall for five minutes with my dad and Marion to see if I felt any better. If not, we would go. Mercifully, as we sat, I got a second wind, allowing me to sit up straight and listen to the band for a couple of hours. I did it by hardly moving, hardly talking and hardly thinking. Then it was a case of eking it out just another 40 minutes and we could all leave together as planned. It had been great to see Mary enjoying herself and dancing. It was the first time I had seen her laughing in a long time and I was grateful my stubbornness had won that at least. The end of the night came. I sat silently on the ride home, itching to keel over on our bed and surrender to sleep. By the time we were halfway home I knew something was wrong.

Sunday July 20 2008. Course 3: Day 9.

This couldn't be right. Dr. Cowdrey said I might not have to go back in until the end of the week. There was no way my counts could be low already? Normally it took around 12 days for them to hit bottom, but here I was feeling awful after only eight. I clung to the belief that I was just feeling off it – sick from the chemo drugs – the thought of going back in already sickened me. But Sunday was a write-off in every sense of the word. I was useless, a wreck. I lay stricken on the sofa slipping in and out of consciousness and vomiting up anything I ate or drunk. I kept telling Mary not to phone the hospital. We were going in the next day for a blood test when they could have me if they wished. But I needed today out, with her. She was fraught with worry and felt complicit in me harming myself. She held the phone at one point but I begged her, even believing I might pick up. Eventually I crawled to bed and passed out, unaware tomorrow would be the beginning of a whole new depth to all this misery.

Monday July 21 2008. Course 3: Day 10.

I was shaking when I woke. I had slept through the night against the odds but clearly something had changed. I felt the cold insidious ebb of an infection gripping me. My counts must have crashed and I had walked straight into some sort of fever. I was hallucinating too my mind throwing big lasso shapes over everything making them seem bigger and rounder. My fingers felt tiny, and I honestly believed I might snap them if I bent or taxed them in some way. I was scared. There was altogether something more urgent, more insistent, more pronounced about this feeling than I had experienced before. The whole treatment so far, and everything associated with it, had had the volume turned up to high.

I pulled on some clothes before collapsing back into bed, exhausted and panting, dragging the covers up to my head. Mary got her things together ready for the trip to hospital, where it was abundantly clear, I would be spending the next couple of weeks. Like a pupil returning after bunking off school, I was expecting a good bollocking for not turning in sooner.

When Mary dropped me off at the entrance an hour later to park up, I could do nothing more than sit in a wheelchair near the door and wait to be pushed to the clinic. Dr. Woodward took one look at me and his smile fell. I never managed one. I wondered whether people ever pass out and fall from a wheelchair. In a side room Dr. Woodward asked about my symptoms and whether I had spoken ahead to the ward. I waffled my explanation, fully aware suddenly how pathetic it sounded. Admissions couldn't just be arranged on the spot, he explained. If I'd have spoken to Durrant Ward last night they could have had a bed ready for me now. As it was, they did not. He seemed pretty mad, albeit in his own very subdued style, like someone railing inside a soundproof bubble. I apologised, shifted position. I tried not to be sick on his desk.

They would have to put me in a bed on EMU, Mary's ward, and begin checking me over until someone could be bumped off of Durrant Ward, hopefully later that day. That sounded fair, I just wanted to be horizontal. Mary pushed me up to EMU where her colleagues had the bed ready for me. I struggled to summon the power to get into it. My blood test was quickly carried out, along with samples for others to see what I had, if it could be identified. It's often the way with infections that the doctors can't be sure exactly what they are treating. They can be more effective if they do, but usually a focussed spectrum of antibiotics is enough to clear it.

My tests quickly returned the verdict we already knew, I was neutropenic, my counts were through the floor, and I had an infection. "Well," I thought. I hadn't hung around getting myself ill this time. I was loaded up on a couple of drugs straight away, given a brief examination by a doctor and put straight on a drip and antibiotic. I spent the next several hours drifting in and out of sleep while Mary sat patiently by my bedside. She still felt responsible for not 'stepping in' as the nurse, intervening, and making me come in earlier. But she was relieved to see me being treated at last. No harm done, hopefully.

I was packed off for a chest X-ray on the way up to Durrant, and was again afraid it was to check, among other things, the cleanliness and functionality of my Hickman line. I knew my doctors wouldn't consider removing it before a last resort, but I still felt nervous about it. Back on Durrant I was wheeled into Side Room 1, the one I'd occupied first. I felt split on just about everything at that point. Was I pleased to be back in hospital or not? Did I feel I was putting too much strain on my mind and body by sticking to September 12? There was little I could say or think about either in that frame of mind that would have been in the least constructive. I was on the mid-point of the roller coaster and there were no station stops.

Tuesday July 22 2008. Course 3: Day 11.

I felt as though I'd wandered into the eye of a storm. Though I did feel pretty wretched, the antibiotics were getting to work, and my health had seemed to find a moment of pause in the middle of all that was going on in my body. I knew I was about to lurch horribly downward on one path or another as though I had momentarily found poise on a rickety tightrope. It was the dizzying wait before the fall. I was already conscious of a parting in my mind. The voices were beginning to talk to me, tell me what to do, chastise me and each other. I was peeling off from reality withdrawing into the recesses of the world I'd discovered during my first course of chemo. I was limited to the bed, where the unseen and unwanted inhabitants of this world seemed to chatter around me. Nothing was ever still. I didn't feel quite at home talking to anybody about the thoughts I was having, often I didn't understand them myself, and so insidious was their creeping I wasn't even sure they were there some of the time. It was a little like a television on in the background. It quietly muttered away, half-noticed, occasionally catching my ear with an observation about my circumstances speaking from somewhere remote. I just couldn't turn it off.

My day was now heavily divided by trips to the toilet. The MACE, famed, I now knew, for its uncompromising effects on the digestive system, had ruined my insides. My stomach still felt scarred and I couldn't eat or drink in any meaningful way, while my bowels were in disarray. I had the all too familiar pain in my backside which was so painful it was affecting all my muscles down there and stopping me passing water. All those things were combining to make me feel pretty miserable indeed. Mary could see this and tried her best to get me thinking positively and focussing on the wedding, on our future. But this was becoming harder and harder for us both.

Wednesday July 23 2008. Course 3: Day 12.

I found myself standing in the bathroom doorway, half-dressed, half awake and something like half-alive. I was gasping, my face was wet. I had no idea if I was headed to or from the toilet but, judging by what looked like a pan full of vomit; I had already paid one visit. My insides were on fire, staging some long overdue protest at their treatment, and I felt sure there was no way they could ever be pacified again. It was some time before I realised the bees must not be real. The swarm had buzzed around me dimming the lights and needling my skin for several minutes, before I even questioned them. The Russian accented commentary was probably in my head too.

I rolled into bed, panting. I had earlier taken a Tamazepam to help me sleep. That now seemed a pointless exercise, though I did manage to duck lightly out of consciousness for odd moments later on. I woke from one doze curled in a ball and shaking. It was rigor, the awful convulsions seeded somewhere between being baking hot and freezing cold. A nurse answered my buzzer and confirmed my temperature had spiked once again. Either the infection I had was presenting itself afresh or a new infection had entered the fray. There was no alternative but to wait out the rigor, which mercifully lasted only 15 minutes or so. But during it I felt acutely alone. Mary always implored me to phone her at any time of the day or night if I needed her and would be upset if I told her in person about some earlier episode during which I hadn't picked up the phone. I wrestled with the idea of disturbing her but decided I would want her to call me. She answered quickly and we talked for a few minutes, during which her main aim was to calm me down. As always, the sound of her voice was enough to bring me back to earth. She came in early that day, and dragged me through possibly the worst 24 hours of my life.

My problems and pains all seemed to come to a head at once. The pain in my backside became so severe I had to consent to a double dose of a painkiller I knew for a fact made me hallucinate. A doctor was bleeped to give me a rectal exam, and, when he arrived, I saw it was the same young man who'd carried out my first, months earlier. During the day my bowels went into free-fall and I managed to soil myself twice. Staff fetched me a pack of man-nappies. My blood tests confirmed I now had a second infection, for which I would need new and different antibiotics. Throughout all this, my pulse was racing. My body felt immersed in shock, deep in the darkest tunnel with no bearing of the light. For the first time I felt truly sorry for myself. I pitied my body, so horribly smashed on the rocks of circumstance. All words of consolation seemed to bounce off me. My positivity, the ocean of belief I had in myself, was lost to me. I felt angry. Bitter. Never yet had I asked 'why' this had to happen. But I felt invaded by doubt, contaminated with it. The very hull of my soul had breached and icy water was coming in. Late at night, when I was alone, I sat and confronted the very real notion that I might not be 'okay'. Everyone assured me I would be. They made me promises. But nobody <u>knew</u> anything. Nobody understood what it was actually like, alone in the dark. I swam for a while in the doubt, looking for any comfort or understanding that might be found there. Then I stopped. I still had the same problems as before. The same assets, I just felt I had betrayed myself, let down those who believed in me. So now what was I going to do?

Thursday July 24 2008. Course 3: Day 13.

"Around 40 per cent of patients don't relapse," Dr. Woodward told me. "They don't need a transplant at all." Those odds seemed tight. It seemed that more than half of those getting a remission would go on to need a transplant based what he'd just said. I tried not to dwell on that thought. Lots of figures were touted about leukaemia and varied depending on who you asked. But I had been thinking about the eventuality of a transplant more and more. The idea of it, of needing one, struck fear into me. It seemed so final recognition of the fact that I was seriously, seriously ill. What if a donor could not be matched? I knew these were fears which would hang over me for as long as I was lucky enough not to relapse. To come through chemotherapy and find it was not enough would be a bitter pill to swallow. "I've spoken to the transplant co-ordinators at Sheffield," Dr. Woodward went on, "and they've said it would be okay for you to have a bone marrow harvest after you've had your fourth course of treatment, if that would be better for your wedding." My eyebrows went up involuntarily. That would buy us some more time and, to my mind, remove the doubt over whether I should have it done. If the bone marrow could be done after the wedding I would definitely go for it. I told Dr. Woodward that that sounded ideal. Decision made.

Friday – Sunday: July 25 – 27 2008. Course 3: Days 14 - 16.

I was well and truly camped in dark territory. My mood, my belief and my spirits had been down for days. I was turning away visitors. I didn't want them to see me in this mess and I didn't have the energy to support any kind of illusion that things were okay. Mary had now completely circumvented traditional visiting hours. She was just there all the time, often late into the night. I didn't have to ask. It was what I needed so she did it without question or complaint.

Course 3 had involved only a five-day course of chemo drugs, but there was nothing to say my counts would return quicker. In fact, Dr. Strong informed me gingerly, in some patients they actually took longer. I faced something like another week of this in all likelihood. This was the Trans-Siberian Express. I was in so much pain and felt so sick, I honestly didn't know if I could take it. For what seemed like the hundredth time I discussed pain relief with Dr. Strong. The strong options were ruled out because they made me insane. Some of the mid-range ones did too or at least made me hallucinate wildly. I preferred the pain to those options. The painkillers I could stand made me constipated, thereby making the problem worse. Nothing really took the edge off the pain anyway it was constantly there draining the joy out of me. I felt I hadn't smiled or laughed in days, and couldn't picture myself ever being happy again. I tried to focus on the wedding, the biggest party of our lives, at the end of all of this, but even that seemed too distant to drag me from the mire in which I found myself. Dr. Strong recognised the change in me; saw that the light had gone out in my eyes. "We could arrange for you to see a psychologist," she said. "Some people find it very useful to talk things through with someone on the outside." I didn't know how I felt about doing that, just tired and daunted which was how I felt about everything that was happening around me. "You're finding it tough, aren't you?" Dr. Strong asked. The words seemed to cut right through me. It was all I could do not to cry. I just nodded. "You're going to have to find a way to get through the days anything that may help you." Her tone softened. "You're an intelligent young man you're going to have to think your way out of this."

Monday July 28 2008. Course 3: Day 17.

It seemed, at last, there had been a breakthrough with my pain relief. The pain varied from day to day anyway; sometimes it was largely bearable, others it reduced me to nothing. But today it was noticeably less severe. I put it down to a new painkiller, Fentanyl, which was administered continuously through a patch. That may well have been helping but Dr. Strong had another explanation. "You have some neutrophils," she said, looking down at my charts. My heart leapt into my mouth. "You had 0.1 yesterday but I didn't want to say anything because one swallow doesn't make a summer. But today you're neutrophils are 1.1." My counts were coming back and sooner than we could have predicted. The neutrophils I had would now be at work repairing where I had pain, fighting infection and generally putting me back together again. In short, the cavalry was here at last.

I had little time to celebrate. "I'm going to ask one of the surgeons to examine you," Dr. Strong went on. "I suspect there might be some underlying problem with your bottom and that's why it's causing you so much pain. There might be something they can do through surgery." I was immediately terrified and my face probably gave as much away. Arse surgery? What had I got myself into now? I exhaled and nodded. If I needed surgery then I needed surgery. I tried to see the positives and not think of words like 'stretching', 'scraping' and 'cutting'. I tried not to think of stitches. Anyway, I might not need surgery at all. There was no point torturing myself until I knew one way or the other. All I knew was this was a problem which had been recurrent and severe. I thought it likely there was something more serious at work. At the very least it would be another bizarre procedure for my ever-growing list. They would be knocking me out, right?

Saturday August 2 2008. Course 3: Day 22.

It was another three days before I had enough platelets in my blood to make surgery an option. My other counts, red and white cells, had come back quickly and strongly, but this time my platelets had really lagged behind. The doctors shrugged. It was normal, they said. It happens. My daily blood tests showed them creeping up, 24, 31, 39. A safe level for surgery is about 50.

I was allowed home for two consecutive nights, returning for a morning blood test to see if we could go ahead. By the Saturday, my body was finally ready to go. I was only just within the range, however, so I was expecting some bleeding. Luckily, the specialist was working the weekend so I was added to the list and told it would probably be that morning. I lay on my bed and waited, staring at the standard issue surgical gown. To say I was apprehensive would be an understatement. I felt like I was on death row. I'd never had a general anaesthetic before. What a place to start. My dad had warned me that I may come round feeling sick, as he always did. I shared his aversion to painkillers so expected to be similarly pre-disposed to sickness as well. But right then that was the least of my worries. I was about to have my backside opened up so a team of experts could have a look-see. I felt sure they would find something, a fissure most likely; the pain was so intense there had to be something.

At 11 o'clock I got word that they were coming to get me. I put on the gown and talked through the consent forms with the nurse, feeling more nervous by the minute. My bed and I were wheeled down to theatre, where I was parked up in some sort of waiting area, before shifting onto one of the operating trolleys. They moved me through to a small room, which

I wasn't sure was the room they'd be operating in or just where the anaesthetic would be administered. I wouldn't get to find out, within two minutes I would be under. I recognised the anaesthetist whom I had met earlier that day. He asked how I was feeling. "Nervous," I replied, guessing that was probably the most common answer he heard. I wondered if he sometimes felt like a magician, a hypnotist putting people to sleep for a living. Keeping them safe from pain. Though I tried not to, I thought of those horror stories of people who are awake during operations but unable to cry out. I thought that I really didn't want to be awake during this one. A canula was put in the back of my hand, and the anaesthetist administered a drug through it. "This will relax you," he said. I put my head back and watched the tick of the clock. That was the last thing I remember.

Far from feeling sick or in pain, I awoke feeling great. I was conscious of talking the nurse's head off as I came round in the recovery area. I was wasted, I soon realised. Whatever I'd been given agreed with me, which made a nice change. I couldn't feel a great deal down below, which I suppose I was thankful for. I was wearing a dressing so ridged and padded it was a little like I'd sat in a child's car seat and couldn't get it off. It was heavily taped to my skin and the hair on the backs of my legs and I knew it would be an ordeal to remove. I settled back, drowsily, as a nurse took me through what the surgeons had found. I had had an ulcer which was surrounded by blood clots. This had been cleaned and any signs of infection were removed. It sounded pretty grim, but I hoped that it might put an end to the pain, at least until my next round of chemo, when it would no doubt flare up again. My surgeon had stipulated that I should stay in overnight for observation, something which I actually didn't mind. That night was Mary's Hen Night and I didn't want to distract her from it in any way. I knew she would be thinking about me and worrying about me anyway, but if I was in hospital being looked after hopefully she'd be able to let go and enjoy herself for a couple of hours. God knows she deserved it.

Sunday August 3 2008. Course 3: Day 23.

The question of how painful it would now be to go to the toilet was answered in the night. It hurt a lot, especially as I had to hurriedly rip off the dressing first. It was a different kind of pain though, and I told myself things would improve in the coming days as I healed. My surgeon, Dr. Guthrie, called by to see me in the morning as I was making arrangements to go home. He explained what he had done in the matter of fact way you might expect from a mechanic when picking up your car from an MOT. I asked the question which was now key, how long do I have to leave before starting chemo again. He smiled. "I can't answer that," he said. "That is something for the haematologists to decide, because I'm not an expert on the effects of chemotherapy. There is nothing to prevent you starting again, as that treatment takes priority, but it may be wise to heal as best you can. But there's nothing to say your problems won't flare up again. That was what I was afraid of. I sensed my doctors wanted me to leave it a while before embarking on Course 4, to ensure I had the best chance of healing properly.

But every day we waited was another day knocked off my recovery for the wedding. If I began Course 4 the following Monday, which was in eight days time, our wedding day would fall on day 33 of the cycle which should be enough time to recover fairly well. Whether my doctors would allow me to start again so soon, or whether there would even be a bed for me, I didn't know. But that was my target and I would be telling my doctors as much.

Dr. Woodward wasn't far behind Dr. Guthrie on his rounds. "When did he say you could begin chemo again?" Dr. Woodward asked. I was afraid he was going to ask me that. "He said it would be down to you." "Aah," he nodded thoughtfully, almost allowing himself a smile, but not quite. "Well then I think the best thing to do would be to see you in clinic on Tuesday and see how you're doing. Then we can discuss when we can get you back in. Your platelets need to come up some more before then. They are still around 50 or 60 and we would like to see a nice meaty one-hundred-and-something before we begin chemotherapy."

My dad and Marion had come in to help me move my things out and once my prescription was ready we headed off, laden with the masses of things I seemed to accumulate when I was in hospital. We huddled into the lift and I caught sight of myself in the mirror. Course 3 had left its scars on me. I had lost most of my body hair and my eyebrows had thinned out a lot. I'd lost almost all of the weight I'd managed to put back on, not to mention the fact I'd needed surgery at the end of it. I reflected on a course that had been every bit as hard as the first. But I'd come through it. It was over, and I was walking out of that hospital on my own two feet. That was an achievement in itself. These were testing times, but I was learning a lot about myself in the process. I saw that, even though at times I fell apart, for the most part, I was stronger than I thought. Perhaps we all are. Self-doubt had always been one of my pet hates just because I believe some people are tougher than they give themselves credit for. Make no mistake, I was dreading Course 4. I was afraid of what it may bring and I knew that it was likely at some point I would crack and tell Mary I couldn't handle it. But more than that I knew I would come through it. In four weeks time, I was going to stand in this very lift carrying my own bags, and know that it was over.

Monday August 4 2008. Course 3: Day 24.

The first days at home were pretty much a non-event. As for the surgery it hurt for me to stand and sitting was out of the question. That left lying down, or more specifically lying on my side, seeing as lying on my back was also painful. I found I was also exhausted, sleeping for a good few hours during the day. My appetite was back, the problem was finding a posture in which I could eat. Though I was hardly an invalid I was very restricted in what I could manage to do. I even had to wear those pads, which was a blow to the ego. Mary chastised me every time I called them nappies but essentially that's what they were.

I felt like a wreck and I was scared to death I would be in a similar state, if not worse, on our wedding day. Mary had said more than once that she would gladly marry me even if I was sitting in a wheelchair. But in my current state I couldn't even manage that. How could you have your ceremony and reception if the only position you could manage was flat out. The answer is that you could not. You would have to call it off. If I could begin the fourth course of treatment before too long then I would have a decent enough recovery time on the other side before the wedding. But when would my doctors allow me to start treatment again? And if I convinced them I was ready before I truly was, might I do myself some lasting damage? There seemed to be no easy decisions to be made in any of this.

Tuesday August 5 2008. Course 3: Day 25.

A fan blew a breeze through the waiting room outside Dr. Strong's office, but did nothing to alleviate the hot flush I was having. They were fairly common at the moment, spells when I would suddenly become unbearably warm. I stripped off my jacket and Marion, who had given me a lift as Mary was seeing her wedding hairdresser, made an attempt at fanning me. I shifted awkwardly on my cushion. I was dosed up on painkillers to get me through the morning, but sitting as I was still disagreed with me. I'd given a blood sample half an hour earlier and I already knew this would reveal a platelet count of more than 100. I knew this by the size of the blood spot visible through the plaster stuck on the crux of my arm. It was small. My blood had clotted and sealed the wound quickly. I'd had enough blood tests in the past few months to establish what I thought was a rough correlation between the size of the blood spot and platelet count. If my counts were all back up, platelets being the hangers-on, then it would be down to Dr. Strong and me when we kicked off again, hopefully for the last time.

When we were called in to Dr. Strong's office she watched me sit, which, again, I did far from happily. I told the truth. I was struggling. It hurt a lot. Dr. Strong nodded, looking through the notes left by the surgeon. "Well," she said, "Dr. Guthrie has written that it would be likely the next course of chemotherapy may need to be delayed." The words bounced hard off my forehead. He had not told me as much in person. "Ordinarily there is no need to get right on with the fourth course," Dr. Strong went on. "We are normally happy to let people have a bit of a break between the last two courses. But obviously we know you have a deadline. Dr. Strong smiled then paused, looking again at my notes. "I was going to say we'll see you in clinic later in the week but I think I could just give you a ring to see how you're recovering. It sounds as though early next week would be the very earliest we could get you in." I agreed. It would be no disaster if I went back in on Wednesday or even Thursday, it would simply be tighter than I would like. But then, it was always going to be.

Since this began we always knew that if we pushed ahead with all the treatment before the wedding I would be affected on the wedding day. It was always a question of how much. But I believed if I could just get there, adrenalin, excitement and determination would get me through the day so that our friends and family might not notice me flagging. I stepped back into the moment, because there was something else that was bothering me. My Hickman line had been hurting me ever since my operation. It looked red and felt really quite sore. When Mary had cleaned it at home, she released a sudden ooze of puss.

To get so far in my treatment and have to have my Hickman line out would be horrible. The end was in sight. I had my theories about what might have happened. The pain was noticeable right after my surgery and I wondered if I had been put in a position which put pressure on the wound. I had no way of knowing and, in a way, it didn't matter. Dr. Strong examined the wound and, to my relief, didn't seem too concerned. She prescribed me an antibacterial cream to apply three times a day and assured me my own neutrophils would also be attacking any infection there. I reminded myself how difficult Course 3 had been. I asked if I could expect similar from Course 4, which would be different drugs again from the dreaded MACE. Dr. Strong forced a smile. "I'm afraid so," she said. "Its high doses of Cytarabine again so it will make you feel sick; but we'll try and get that under control from the start this time." "Yes, please," I replied, but I had heard that before.

Saturday August 9 2008. Course 3: Day 29.

Because it seemed like my only chance to do so, I invited some close friends round to mine on Saturday for a pseudo Stag do. I had my reservations about doing this. Firstly, of course, I was worried about my health. Since I'd been out there had been good days and bad days. On the latter, I felt exhausted, in pain and capable of very little. I didn't want my friends to see me that way. Secondly, I didn't know how others would behave around me. Would they feel guilty about drinking if I didn't feel like it? When we went out, historically, this crowd didn't do things by halves. I didn't want to be the one putting a dampener on my own night. I knew that, ultimately, every one of them knew the score and would understand if the night imploded, but that didn't stop me worrying about it. Some of my friends, I suspected, didn't comprehend just how ill I was. For them, I wanted to keep it that way by smiling, looking well and, if necessary, lying.

As it turned out I was okay. The night was fairly subdued but I did struggle a little with tiredness. I went for a lie-down several times during proceedings, but these were all short enough that nobody noticed. But some of the lads asked if I wanted to head into town later on and I had to say I didn't really feel up to it. We stayed in, then, played some cards until about 2 a.m. That was plenty late enough for me. I was exhausted and spent the whole next day in bed.

Monday August 11 2008. Course 3: Day 31.

I got out of the car and looked up at the windows of Durrant Ward. The previous evening I had received the call saying there was a bed for me, and everything became very real again. I had jumped straight from Course 2 into Course 3 and here I was about to plough into number four with hardly a break to speak of. But this was what I had wanted, what we had agreed. It didn't make it easier though. I couldn't say hand on heart that I felt ready to start again. I couldn't say I had recovered from my operation adequately to make beginning chemo again sensible, but time was against us and I knew what I was getting into. I was fighting leukaemia. If I was going to beat it I was in for a scrap. So be it. This was what it was all about. This was what it took to beat it. You had to steel yourself a thousand times against every infection, every re-admission, every lonely night on the ward, every drug they pumped into you that you knew would make you more ill. "Be a man," I told myself, "one more time."

Course 4

Tuesday August 12 2008. Course 4: Day 1: Chemo Day 1.

We wasted little time in getting started on the MidAC course of drugs which comprised an inky blue chemical called Mitoxantrone and what Dr. Cowdrey called 'industrial' doses of my old friend Cytarabine. It was the latter, or more its high dosage, which would cause me the problems of sickness, I was warned. At least this course only required me to be hooked up to a drip for five hours a day. Five hours, five days; and then goodness willing, no looking back. I could be free of all this.

It was important, I felt, to be proactive from the off and we agreed to start me on the full gamut of anti-sickness drugs. I felt that last time the damage had been done to my stomach before we got a grip of it. I also asked for the diet supplement, Calogen, from the beginning to try and minimise weight loss. I was put on eye drops too, as the high dose Cytarabine was known to cause conjunctivitis. The only other thing I had on prescription was food. Mary was now bringing me in my afternoon and evening meals as I just couldn't stomach hospital food any more. The last thing I wanted to do was be seen as snobbish about what the caterers served, in fact during the early months of my treatment I had defended it. I had just reached a wall with it and couldn't go any further. Imagine your worst memories of school dinners with the cuisine re-boiled a couple of times and you're somewhere close to imagining how it tasted to me at that time. My taste hadn't returned to normal and what I fancied to eat could vary a great deal from minute to minute, so I simply couldn't find anything on the hospital menu I felt able to eat. Trying to force down something unappetising just made me sick. Most of the time I got by on sandwiches and didn't feel like tackling hot meals. If Mary, and on occasion Marion, hadn't catered, I don't know what I would have done. Go hungry most likely.

Going back into chemo seemed to get harder each time. Coming through the nightmare of Course 3 had been a real trial and, now my health had returned, the thought of becoming ill again was simply heartbreaking. The whole process felt like getting behind the wheel of a car and being ordered to crash into a brick wall, smashing my body to pieces, then repeating the cycle once I'd been nursed back to health. Here I was again, strapping myself in for another RTA, but this was tempered with the promise that it could be for the last time. Once more unto the breach.

Wednesday – Saturday: August 13 – 16 2008. Course 4: Days 2 - 5: Chemo Days 2 - 5.

What a summer of sport to tantalise the retinas. For Course 1 I got to watch my team win the FA Cup, albeit in a stupor, Course 2 ran alongside the European Championships, though England were sadly absent. Now, Course 4 was to be graced with the richest bonanza of them all, the Olympics, day-long coverage of the most sublime and bizarre sporting action the world had to offer was here to save my sanity. I had five days to get through on the chemo drugs. To be unconscious for it all was preferable but never offered, so staring at the TV in a semi-coma for eight hours a day seemed like a reasonable alternative. Team GB's best medal haul in decades meant I had plenty of 'our own' to cheer on, but I was equally happy watching the banal ballets play out between Algerian Tae Kwon Do hopefuls or Quiff-haired fencers from Belgium. No matter how welcomingly diverting the on-screen action became, however, there was no banishing the sickness. The anti-emetics were definitely helping, I would hate to attempt chemo without them, but a good portion of queasiness is always destined to get through. This was tolerable though managed better than it had been thus far in my treatment. I found once the sickness and vomiting began it was hard to banish. This time I had been started on the full complement of anti-sickness drugs from the start and I had managed to keep eating and keep something in my stomach at all times to minimise the horrible acidic feeling in my insides.

Undergoing chemo was no different to anything else; you could get better at it. I felt early on that this course might be kinder to me, at least more so than Courses 1 and 3. With what I had learned about my body to date, and what the doctors had learned about me, maybe we could close out on a high. To get through without infection was still a pipe-dream, but achievable none-the-less.

Day 5 came and I had my final bag of Mitoxantrone hooked up. I watched it snake down the wire into my veins and told myself this could be the last dose of chemo I would need. Finito. Later on Dr. Cowdrey stopped by with the result of my blood tests. "Your counts are okay," he told me, "but they seem to be coming down steadily." I didn't know if he would agree to let me out at all after last time, "lesson learned", I beamed to him, telepathically. "Your counts came down so quickly last course," he mused, tossing his head to either side, "It's hard to predict what will happen this time." *Bismillah, let me go.* "I think we should see you in clinic on Wednesday for another test. But bring some things with you as we may need to admit you there and then, depending on results." I nodded gratefully. He'd just given me four days outside of the box. Few greater gifts are ever bestowed.

Sunday – Wednesday: August 17 – 20 2008. Course 4: Days 6 - 9.

Being on the outside felt like being in the eye of the storm. We seemed to be waiting, rather than enjoying it, but we did use the time to tie up some of the loose ends for the wedding. Once again Mary and I seemed to keep falling victim to the other's moods, feeling rarely happy and positive at the same time. I remember on one occasion trying to cheer her up by telling her, in fact, how lucky we were, and I illustrated this by talking about the plight of people in Afghanistan. That went down very badly indeed. But if we were both secretly keen to get back on the hospital hamster wheel we didn't have long to wait.

On the Wednesday we made our way into clinic with some of my things, as instructed, should my counts show I needed to be admitted. We found the clinic busier than ever and kept catching sight of Drs. Cowdrey and Woodward bouncing around like moths in a bell-jar trying to get round to everyone. We waited a couple of hours before there was even chance to take some blood from me, then another 45 minutes for the result. Dr. Cowdrey called me in to his office and confirmed I was neutropenic, shattering a fragile hope I had of being sent away for another day or two, and my old hang-out of Side Room 4 was ready for me up on Durrant Ward.

What happened next is something of a nightmarish blur. Some parts I remember well, others I have no recollection of. Then there are the bits I recall which didn't actually happen. The speed of my decline still frightens me. I walked onto the ward with a smile and less than 72 hours later my family were called in to say their goodbyes.

Thursday August 21 2008. Course 4: Day 10.

I began feeling unwell in the afternoon on the day following my admission. I knew an infection was taking hold, its beginnings were similar to others I'd had while neutropenic. I told Dr. Woodward when he called in to see me that I could feel the beginnings of an infection, a subtle stir in my wellbeing, something not quite as it should be. He looked at my notes, "Well you haven't spiked a temperature yet, so let's see how it plays out." I could have been wrong, but I didn't think so. I'd felt this way enough times to know what happened next. But until he knew what he was dealing with, Dr. Woodward couldn't just start throwing antibiotics at it. He was to get his answer soon enough.

Friday August 22 2008. Course 4: Day 11.

My temperature began to go up and I was beginning to feel pretty rotten and very tired. While Mary sat in the chair beside me, I fell into a troubled sleep. I awoke some hour or so later and knew immediately I was going to be sick. The toilet may as well have been in France, as close as it was, I wasn't going to get there. I jumped to my feet, plunged one of them onto the pedal of the bin and was sick, quite violently, into it. Mary, for whom this outburst must have been a little startling, rushed to my side while I continued emptying my stomach into the bin. I must have told her I was okay; because she went to get me some of those charming cardboard sick bowls were I to be sick again. I began to feel distinctly like something was sinking in my chest. I became aware I was suddenly sitting on the toilet and Mary was trying to help me up. But my legs and arms were not my own. They felt rubbery and heavy, too heavy for me to move. The weight of my torso took itself forward, making a bid to smash my paralysed bulk into the floor. Mary was all that stopped this from happening, by simply putting herself in the way to bounce me back upright. I remember her repeating my name and the word "No" with such a fear in her voice that I knew something was seriously wrong. My legs were shaking violently. I heard "No" once more and blacked out.

The next thing I remember was lying flat in bed, my head was being held to one side. I had been sick again and a matron held a suction pump in my mouth to ensure I didn't choke. I could hear the rapid beep of the heart-rate monitor, and Dr. Woodward's voice saying, "So it definitely isn't a cardiac arrest?" Someone answered him: "No." I was aware of several bodies around the bed but couldn't look up. This was the crash team and, why were they talking about heart attacks? I later learned the infection had caused my blood pressure to drop through the floor, making me black out. For the time being, however, I was confused and didn't know what was going on. Mary was one of those faces surrounding my bed and she looked genuinely terrified. My little episode had worried staff enough to ship me over to the High Dependency Unit, a ward where patients could be given round-the-clock care. It's where you went when they needed to keep an eye on you, and the ratio of patients to staff was roughly 1:1.

I was wheeled into one of the unit's sickrooms. I was still neutropenic, not to mention carrying some nasty infection, so it was as well to keep me separate from everyone else. Once in HDU, my condition began to stabilise, thanks to medication to regulate my blood pressure. My pulse was still racing, however, and showed no signs of slowing down. It was an uneasy afternoon, but my stats were settled, albeit not in the ranges they should be. Mary had already told me she was staying with me overnight, though I had urged her to go home and rest.

At around 10 p.m. she left my side for five minutes to call down to the EMU, where she worked, to talk to her boss. Soon after she left something changed. My head began to swim with dizziness and I felt the same sinking feeling again, as though my mattress was sucking me in like a snake with its oversized prey. I was fading fast and needed help. I searched weakly for the buzzer to summon the nurses. It was on the wall several feet away, which I knew I would never reach in time. I opened my mouth to shout for help. The words limped out, muted by my malaise and confusion. I tried again. "Help," I shouted, but my voice was cracked and slurred. I looked out of the partition window to the nurses' station to see if anyone had heard me. Nobody moved. I blacked out again.

In the end it was Mary who found me. She returned to find me unconscious, eyes writhing in the back of my head. The crash team were called and the scene played out much as before. I came round to see the now-familiar crew around my bed. I blinked. They smiled. "I need to tell you something," I said, suddenly, purposefully. "Is Mary here?" "No, she's outside," one of the matrons said. She had been shepherded to safe distance when the crash team moved in. "Good," I nodded weakly. "Because I don't want her to know." The matron leaned in, "What is it? What's wrong?" "Okay, but you can't tell her. You can't tell her that I've spent all the wedding money." All the faces around the bed looked ahead blankly. No-one seemed to know what to say. Was this confused rambling or the confession of a guilty groom? "It's gone. I've spent all the wedding ... erm ... what do you call it?" "Money," one chimed in helpfully. "Yes," I said, eyes closed. "The budget is bust. I had to spend it all on this chemotherapy-whatsit." Though I clearly remember saying all that, I'm not sure where it came from. A combination of drugs and confusion. Our budget was still intact as far as I knew. It might now remain untouched altogether; if my health did not improve quickly there would be no wedding at all.

Saturday August 23 2008. Course 4: Day 12.

Mary had stayed the night with me, now terrified to leave me unattended. I'd proved I couldn't be trusted not to conk out. Neither of us had much sleep to speak of. By the morning, I looked pretty terrible. My face was bright red and swollen. My stomach, too, looked inflated and had become very bloated and painful. My feet had all but doubled in size. One of the nurses told Mary that tests on my blood had revealed I had contracted ESBL, a so-called 'superbug' in that it actually feeds on certain types of antibiotics. It is in the same family in that respect as MRSA and C-diff, the infection that had caused outbreaks in both hospitals in which I'd been treated. I'd spent so much time worrying about and dodging C-diff that one of its relatives had snuck up on me.

Mary didn't feel it was necessary that I knew what I had just at that moment. She commented that I already looked scared that morning, and hearing that I had a superbug and was bang in trouble wouldn't have been helpful. The problem was that, to treat the ESBL I needed to be given the antibiotic Imepenem, which I had demonstrated during my first course of treatment that I happened to be allergic to. I had reactions to members of the penicillin family of antibiotics, ranging from a rash to becoming hot and feverish if I had them. There was little choice, however, Imepenem was the only drug effective in treating ESBL, and I was going to need an awful lot of it, direct to my veins.

First I was given a dose of steroids intravenously to help boost my body's defences. Then the antibiotics were pushed through my Hickman line. It didn't go well. I vomited and blacked out again.

The crash team were called. If they had some kind of loyalty scheme I would be racking up some serious air miles. But this time wasn't like the others. I wasn't waking up. My heart beat was sky high and I just wasn't responding to anything. Mary was asked to leave the room. What happened during those next minutes, I don't know. They must have worked hard to keep me here, but still I was unresponsive. Essentially, I was slipping away. My heart was under so much strain it could have easily given out. I had youth on my side, maybe, and a fierce drive to live, especially after coming this far, if that could be said to count for anything. But I was weak. My body had slogged through four rounds of chemo, two in rapid succession, and those were not the ideal precursors for facing a bug of this gravity.

A doctor briefed my dad, Marion and Mary, telling them things were looking bleak. It was as well they came back in to say their goodbyes should the worst happen. With every passing second that eventuality looked more and more like the only outcome. For my family, this was the bitterest pill they could have been asked to swallow, after travelling with me for the nightmarish past four months. To have witnessed every freefall, shared every small triumph along the way, only for me to be taken now. We were so close to the end. This would surely be the cruellest deal of all, for my fiancée especially, just weeks from our wedding. What sour horror would then await her on the day that should have been the happiest of her life. When the doctor told her the score, she says that she 'howled'. People can and do fall apart at such times. Had roles been reversed it would have been the end of my world. I'm not sure I could have summoned the strength to do anything.

But what my girl did next is the single most inspiring thing I could name. When her back is to the wall she is a street fighter, and so much stronger than she would credit to herself. If you've ever heard the expression 'rage against the dying of the light' you'll understand.

Rather than quietly implode in a drab little room in the hospital, rather than do as she'd been told and say "I love you. Goodbye." She did something else. She barged past the doctor and back into the room where I lay somewhere between death and life. She fought to her place at the side of my bed and began, for want of a better description, to shout at me for being so utterly selfish. "Richard," she bellowed, "don't you dare. Come back to us. You need to fight it and wake up." My dad and Marion, who had now joined the crowd in the room, began to do the same, calling me back to life. Drugs and technology had done what they could for me. I'd had the science, now I needed some magic. The three of them called to me, and from somewhere deep underground I heard them. I was conscious on some level, but I was lost, dazed and dizzy somewhere far off. Then I heard her voice, telling me what I needed to do. The tone was stern, angry almost, a tone I'd awakened more times than perhaps I should have in the past. A lifetime ago. I knew the undertones, I was to do as I was told. I can remember vividly what it was like, drifting away from the world. There were no lights, to go towards, or otherwise, no angelic singing. Not for my sort anyway. It was like sinking into something thick, thick enough to pin my limbs to my side so I was swallowed all the faster. How apt that should be the way to go, mimicking the draining nightmares that were a fixture of what sleep I had. Always black, but I could feel myself sinking past level after level of something. I felt placid, however, as if this was all there had ever been.

I have no doubt in my mind that I would have died had I not heard Mary's voice. It opened some internal floodgate and the memories began to gush in, memories of who I had been. "Richard, you need to wake up." I knew then what I had to do, and something very determined took over. A swell of something like anger began throbbing in my chest and the sinking slowed, ever-decreasing until it stopped. Then I began to rise, kicking my way up from the bottom of the ocean towards the air. The levels I had passed on the way down were racing by me as I ascended and each one seemed to claw at me as I went, ripping shreds of my arms. I became aware of the burning pain in my chest as I climbed. The pain only grew more intense the higher I went, but I knew I had to kick on to the source of it. There was a flash bulb of light as I opened my eyes, the brightest I had ever seen.

I have no memory of what I am told I did next, which was to sit up and pull the long tube of the ventilator, which had been breathing for me, out of my throat. Surrounding me must have been a dozen people. I squinted at them, surveying the reddened eyes of my family. Even one of the nurses, a friend of Mary's, was crying. My dad just kept saying to me, "Well done," over and over. Mary looked as though she had just let go of the weight of the world. She gripped my hand. What have I missed, I wondered. What was everyone so down about? A doctor asked me how I felt, was I in any pain? I drowsily stopped to think, realising my heart felt as though it was on fire, beating so fast my pulse felt like a continuous drone. The pain took my breath. "My chest," I said, clutching it. "My heart." A couple of the doctors shot each other a look which I intercepted, and it told me I was still in a world of trouble. One of them said the word 'Morphine'. I mumbled something about my sanity's aversion to it, and was told rather sternly that I would be taking a stiff dose straight away.

My family were ushered out of the room once again. My dad clutched my foot as he passed. "Well done," he said again, hand clenched as though cheering his son's crucial goal from the sidelines. I still wasn't sure what I'd done exactly. I sat there still, while my bed spun and faceless people fussed around, until the doctor and my family returned. "Listen, Richard," the doctor said, "you are very poorly at this moment in time. We're doing what we can to get this bug but we can't have you keep having these blackouts. You need all your strength to fight this. You will probably soon find it harder to breath. What I am proposing we do is to put you on a ventilator and put you to sleep for a few days. That way we can control your blood pressure and stop you having these attacks. I blinked, still very confused about what was going on. Everyone wore the same mask of concern. Things were worse than I feared. What choice did I have? I nodded my agreement. The doctors clearly felt I might not be so lucky should I black out again. I overheard that I was having an antibiotic 'blue-lighted' over from Nottingham. That is to say ferried by an ambulance, siren screaming all the way.

True to the doctor's word I was finding it very hard to breath. My lungs felt tight and painful, and I was constantly short of breath, even when wearing the oxygen mask. One of the nurses brought in the solution. She called it the hood, but I would come to know it as the bubble. We had a love-hate relationship from the start. The bubble was a small plastic chamber not much bigger than my head. This was significant because it was my head which would be living in it for the foreseeable future. In the bottom was a hole with an elasticated rim. This would form a seal around my neck once my head had wriggled through. Oxygen would be delivered into the bubble via a tube which attached to the side. The pressure inside the bubble combined with the clever valve on the side to help the wearer breath. Essentially, when I began to breathe in, air would be pushed into my lungs helping them to inflate fully with only half the effort. That all sounded great, only I was not a fan of enclosed spaces. I wouldn't say I was claustrophobic; I just didn't like being boxed in for long periods of time. When I first put the bubble on, I found it very difficult to relax and breathe naturally. This was because of a natural instinct not to breathe re-cycled air. For example, I wouldn't put my head in a carrier bag, seal it around my neck, and feel comfortable about breathing for very long. This is exactly what it felt like, and it took a while to divorce myself from the idea that I was breathing bad air. When I did manage to calm myself, I could breathe much more easily.

A clip attached to my finger monitored the levels of oxygen in my blood. In a healthy person with good lung function, this should read around 98-100%. With no breathing apparatus at all, my reading would quickly slip down to the low 80s and the monitor would beep a warning. I would be asked to kindly put the bubble back on. Then there were the logistical problems of wearing such a thing. It got hot inside, so that when removed a mixture of water vapour and sweat would trickle down my neck. I would get itches on my head and face I was unable to scratch, and I felt like one of those dogs with a protective cone around its head. When wearing the bubble I was as good as deaf. I would see my visitor's lips moving but could make out nothing of what they were saying; all I could hear was one exaggerated breath after another. It was like being trapped in a lift with *Darth Vader*. But there was one definite benefit to the bubble being brought into the equation it meant that my stats had levelled off sufficiently to put the doctors off putting me to sleep. They felt I had a good enough chance of beating it with my eyes open.

Sunday August 24 – Monday September 1 2008. Course 4: Days 13 - 21.

There was a war on. At least, in my head there was. Soldiers would troop past my bedside, some with horrific wounds, a recently severed arm, a dangling eyeball. Others would whisper in my ears in foreign tongues. In fact, the upper corner of my room had been blown away, destroyed in a bombing raid. Stranger than all of this, was that I found none of it the least bit strange. A Russian paratrooper stumbled past me one day dragging his parachute and cradling his leaking guts. I wished him a good morning. It was a few days before I twigged that I was under the spell of some pretty convincing hallucinations. That's the thing about being crazy you have no idea that you're actually tripping out. You can be nuttier than squirrel shit and something outrageous taking place before your eyes feels rather mundane. These visions were no doubt a combination of my sepsis and medication, but quite what made them take the form they did I couldn't say.

Sometimes I would utter something so off-the-wall and irrelevant that Mary could only stare back at me. It must be a frightening thing to watch. But for the most part I was inhabiting the same world as everyone else. The problem was it felt like a pretty miserable place to be. Never had I looked, felt or indeed been, so ill. My hair and eyebrows were a distant memory; my arms were blue with bruises from failed attempts to get canulas into my collapsed veins. I now had a central line in my neck through which drugs were administered. That, in addition to my Hickman line, canulas in my right arm and left foot, a heart-rate monitor cable on my chest and an O_2 level detector on my finger meant I had six different wires coming out of me. Seven if you counted my IPod. Then, of course, there was the matter of the bubble over my head. I felt more machine than man. I was suffering from terrible bloatedness and was hardly eating or sleeping. I was forbidden from leaving my bed, but found having to use a bedpan very demeaning. I remember having a fairly heated exchange with a nurse in which I asked several times to be allowed to cross the ward to the toilet. Several times, I was refused. I felt extremely low and would often just burst into tears without a moment's notice.

Mary and my dad would try to lift my spirits by promising me that in a week or so I might be well enough to go back to Durrant Ward. But even they knew that was no comfort, it felt like being forced to put my hand on a hot stove and then being told, "don't worry, in a week or so you can take it off." Every second on that ward burned a little deeper. It dragged and there was no opportunity for respite. Mary and her Mum would sit with me through the nights and I was thankful for their presence, which at times felt like the only thing keeping me tethered to my sanity. I was convinced an enormous beetle waited under my bed for me to be left alone. Everything seemed to be the wrong size, as though every fixture of reality had passed through a hallucination filter. My body had changed its proportions too, but I wasn't imagining that part. My ankles, feet and abdomen were painfully and surreally swollen. My navel, hitherto an 'inny', had ballooned into an 'outy'. Despite retaining all this water, I was hardly passing any. It wasn't until days later that I began to purge it all and how. My fluids were monitored by a balance sheet. Everything I drank was documented, along with everything I deposited in the bottles provided. A normal person would, of course, drink a fair bit more than they passed over the course of the day. But in one day alone I shed a couple of litres more than I drank once it began to come off. Being bed-ridden probably contributed in no small part to this swelling.

All-in-all, I didn't leave the bed for ten days straight. That's a stretch for anyone, including the terminally lazy. I'm in the other camp. I'm a fidget who hates being cooped up. The days slid by at an agonising crawl. There was little I could do to amuse or distract myself, as I felt too rotten to do anything. When you are that low you don't even have it in you to read. I had to keep asking for the television to be turned off because the inane chatter was more than I could cope with. When you've been reminded so vividly of your mortality, watching people witter on about the different ways cardboard cut-out celebrities are wearing neck scarves leaves you a little cold. Part of me wanted to storm their film sets and plead with them to recognise how utterly trivial it all was. But that's the way of things. We happily immerse ourselves in the white noise of modern living until the savage simplicity of it all slaps us on the forehead. I felt truly desperate.

I was being given GCSF injections, a growth hormone designed to stimulate my bone marrow into producing the cells I desperately needed to start kicking into the infection. I had been given slowly incrementing doses of Imepenem, the antibiotic that fights off ESBL, because I was believed to be allergic to it. The dosage was upped after I appeared to be desensitised to it. It seemed to be working. I was stabilising, but all I could think of was getting out of that room, off that ward. That's no criticism of the staff who worked there; it just feels like death's waiting room. I was comfortably the youngest person on the ward and felt, for whatever reason, I didn't belong there. I wasn't in the same league as this lot, surely? The uncomfortable truth was that I was. I'd come pretty close to checking out. It was a reminder of how serious my disease was. Albeit it was not the leukaemia which had put me on the brink, rather the treatment itself, but the fact remained. People died from what I had. Lots of them. I was largely powerless in it all.

Dr. Cowdrey would come down to see me sporadically, but always carrying a very serious expression. I'd become accustomed to his smile, and he mine, as we discussed matters grave and serious. Though I tried to keep up my end of the bargain, Dr. Cowdrey looked very sombre indeed which only served to deflate me a little further. I was feeling better and itching to return to Durrant Ward, particularly as I would have my own toilet there. Dr. Cowdrey did make passing references to getting me back there, but not for a few days and only then if a side room was available. I asked about the wedding date, now less than three weeks away, and if it was likely I could recover by then. "Yes, I still think so," Dr. Cowdrey said. For now though I couldn't walk, or didn't expect I would be able to anyway. But how I longed to try.

It was a few more days of long, drawn-out nothingness before I was given permission to attempt crossing the ward on foot to the toilet. With Mary on one side and a nurse on the other, we collectively manoeuvred my feet round to the side of the bed, and, as I sat up, to the floor. My legs felt very weak and alien but as I pushed against them they did not buckle. I allowed more of my weight to come forward and still they pushed back. With quite a bit of help, I stood for the first time in ten days. My balance was unsure but with my two chaperones clutching my elbows I was able to shuffle slowly towards the door. It was hard to believe something so mundane, so totally underestimated, could be so exhilarating. Just to shift into a different point of view galvanised my soul and I dared to believe, more than ever, that everything was going to be okay.

Tuesday September 2 2008. Course 4: Day 22.

After ten days on the High Dependency Unit I was released to go back to Durrant Ward. This was the home straight. I had packed in the four rounds of chemo before the wedding. I was grateful to my doctors for getting me there, as they'd promised. My treatment was over. With any luck I would be sorted, free to re-join the world. I was still weak and my counts were sluggish, but I felt in a day or two I would be well enough to leave. I set myself the target of two days to be out of there. Mary and the rest of my family warned me not to overburden myself; after all little more than a week ago they were saying their goodbyes to me. But after the stint in HDU I couldn't wait to get out, to get back to being me. I'd missed so much already.

After a couple of days-worth of antibiotics on Durrant Ward, my temperature had stayed down long enough for Dr. Cowdrey to be satisfied I could leave. I hit my target, as it turned out. I think some of my family thought this was premature, but Dr. Cowdrey wasn't going to put me at any risk. He's a humanist, he recognises the importance to the mental wellbeing of patients that going home serves. I shunned a wheelchair and walked out of there, which was always important to me. After all that had gone before I expected to feel a sense of elation at leaving, but I felt strangely numb. It was almost as if I didn't really believe that this was the end of it all.

Had I fared better in Course 4, there would have been the real possibility of being selected for a fifth course of chemo in the medical trials I was part of. As it turned out, what with Course 4 nearly killing me and all, Dr. Cowdrey pulled the plug. Putting me straight into more chemo would probably have finished me off. The chances were that it might not make a difference either. I had achieved remission after Course 1 so by now there shouldn't be any cancerous cells remaining in my body. Dr. Cowdrey even told me in some trials they were even questioning the necessity of a fourth course. I had to raise an eyebrow at that, but the way I saw it, if there was this malignancy growing inside me, I didn't want to tickle it, I wanted it nuked. Obliterated. I couldn't entertain the idea of it coming back.

My dad told me that, when I was in HDU, I told him the first thing I was going to do when I got out was buy a gun. If the leukaemia returned, I said, I was going to shoot myself in the head. I have no memory of this, but it tells you exactly how I felt at the time. It's not like me to surrender like that. If it did come back, I would find a way to pick myself up and get back in the ring. I was in a dog-fight and I couldn't imagine a time when I would just tap out. If not for myself, for Mary. I'd promised I would never leave her. I loved her so completely, so hopelessly, and that was bigger than cancer. It would never, ever crack us. I felt I was more likely to live for ever than die like that. I didn't consider myself brave, just brave enough. And that stems entirely from her. She's the reason to win.

Friday September 5 2008. Course 4: Day 25.

It didn't take long for us to realise that something was still wrong with me. For the first couple of days at home I felt more or less okay, in line with where I'd been at least. But I was feeling weaker each day rather than stronger. I would drift between very hot and very cold and had the shakes. Despite all that had gone before, I couldn't lose the "I'll probably feel better tomorrow" attitude. This was born of my fear of going back into hospital. It paralysed me.

We were a week from the wedding and I couldn't face being told there was something wrong. In the end, Mary phoned the ward and Dr. Cowdrey, inevitably, asked me to come in. I took a bed on EMU, Mary's ward, and waited for him to arrive. I still believed he would tell me this was natural and I would be okay after a day or two's rest. But, first off, he had another theory. After listening to my symptoms, he asked what medication I was still taking. The only thing I had been on recently was the Fentanyl patch, a painkilling drug absorbed slowly through the skin, but I had stopped taking it a few days earlier. "How long had you been on that?" he asked. I thought about it. "A couple of months, ten weeks perhaps." The ghost of a smile flashed across Dr. Cowdrey's face. "It may be," he said, "that you're withdrawing. I can't be sure of that. We need to do some blood cultures to check there isn't something else going on, but it sounds as though you may be going 'cold turkey'". I grinned. It was a relief to learn that the problem may be no more serious than my being a drug addict. The nurse managed, eventually, to get some blood out of my collapsed veins, characteristic of a drug addict, don't you think? The cultures were sent off but, for the time being, I was to stay in hospital until the results were back.

The real problem, it turned out, was that I had e-coli. When Dr. Cowdrey broke this news to me, I didn't take it particularly well. He said what he thought most likely was that the ulcer in my backside that was operated on, had somehow resurfaced and was releasing bugs into my blood stream. That or something in the region of the bowel. I would most likely need another operation to stop it just coming back periodically. I was inconsolable at this news. My target and focus through all of this had been the wedding and, as such, had become something of a holy grail. My determination to get there had become an obsession. To be told, in the week it was due to take place, that we may have to postpone was extremely hard to take. I felt like someone had died.

I phoned my dad to tell him but couldn't even bring myself to say the words. I had to pass the phone to Mary. I was started on the course of antibiotics again to combat the infection, and an appointment was scheduled for me to see Dr. Guthrie, the surgeon who had operated on me the last time.

Saturday September 6 2008. Course 4: Day 26.

I paced about in my room, absolutely distraught, more fragile than I had felt in my whole life. In my mind, the wedding would have to be called off. The one thing we'd both pinned our hopes on was sliding out of view, being eaten by the cancer like everything else. Its parting shot at me really stung. I felt so furious at myself I wanted to leap out of the window. Mary had to come in long before visiting time to try and calm me down. We would always prop each other up when needed; countering one person's doubts with the strongest arm the other could muster. It must have been hard for her to summon that belief when she probably felt the same way I did. But, at my lowest point, as a hundred times before, she carried me.

I was soon summoned to Dr. Guthrie's outpatient clinic, and waited with the haunted expression only a person who's queued for a rectal exam can appreciate. When he called me in, Dr. Guthrie didn't seem too sure why I was there, other than for a routine follow-up. I explained the problem and the possible cause suggested by my doctors. To my relief, Dr. Guthrie didn't buy it. "I wouldn't have thought that likely," he said, "but let's examine you and see what's what."

My head began to spin with possibilities. If my old problem wasn't to blame for the e-coli, what was? If it couldn't be identified then what was to stop it returning? More pressing than these, however, was exactly how I would be undergoing an exploratory procedure inside my arse while fully conscious. The answer, as would soon be made clear to me, was with a unique piece of equipment. Now, I've mulled over a few different ways of describing it, but couldn't get passed 'a dildo with a camera on it'. I didn't get too good a look at the little fella, but would have been happier had it been smaller. There must have been some sort of light incorporated because, well, you need a torch if you're going caving, don't you.

I was ordered onto the bed, where, stripped below the waist, I had to curl up in a foetal position on one side. "This is all we did with you last time," Dr. Guthrie said, "only it would have been too painful for you at the time without a general anaesthetic." Too right, and now? Dr. Guthrie assured me that he would be gentle, before lubeing up a digit. In the end, the procedure wasn't too bad, largely because Dr. Guthrie knew what he was doing. "Well," he said, "I'm really pleased with how that has healed. There's no sign of infection." I was relieved. Though I wanted the cause to be identified, I didn't want that to be it. Dr. Guthrie was going to write up some notes and then speak to my doctors, who I assumed would be sent back to square one.

When they came to see me later they were a little perplexed. Dr. Woodward said he still thought their theory was the most likely explanation, but they would just press on with the antibiotics and get the infection cleared. We were fast running out of time, though. The wedding was just four days away, and Dr. Cowdrey was suggesting something in the region of nine days-worth of antibiotics. That clearly presented a problem. I talked it through with Dr. Cowdrey, and we both believed there was a way. "What we could do," he said, "is continue with the antibiotics up until the night before the wedding, and then you can go home. But you will need to come back in first thing for a double dose of antibiotics, then another double dose about midday. Then we won't need to see you until first thing the morning after." I could have kissed him. I would need the antibiotics every eight hours. So, after I was sent home, I would need to return to hospital three times each day for about a week. The fact I would have to leave at the crack of dawn the morning after the wedding stung Mary a bit. I wasn't mad about the idea either but it was preferable to the alternative. I would ask my dad to take me, at around 6 a.m., then we could comfortably be back early enough for a snooze before breakfast.

The only problem, it seemed, was exactly how I was going to be strong enough to get through the wedding. I felt really weak, mostly because my red cells were still low. But Dr. Cowdrey had the answer to that too. I would have three bags of blood transfused two days before the wedding, as they generally take that long to perk up a person's counts. I needed them badly.

My dad picked up my suit from the hire place and brought it in for me to try it on. Just putting it on was draining and I had to keep sitting down. It made me think, yet again, about the miracle of giving blood. Three strangers would make the difference between my wedding day being a circus side-show or all we dreamed it could be. And they'll never know it.

Our Wedding Day

**Friday
September 12 2008.
Course 4: Day 32.**

The five smartly-dressed sentries around my bed at dawn turned out to be the best men and ushers' suits hanging on a costume rail. The clock said 4.59 a.m. I deactivated the alarm before it had its moment of glory, for which it had waited, purposefully, and without sound all night. Seemed cruel really, but I needed just a few moments more of silence. I'd been released the evening before and a handful of mates and family had stayed over with me after a night on the Wii. We had finally crawled into our beds, sofas or stretches of carpet, at around 2 a.m. I heard my sister's boyfriend's alarm go off across the hall, and Dave uttered the groan of a man to whom life has just dealt a particularly petty blow. I had to stifle a laugh. He had the short straw of driving me into hospital at that ungodly hour for my first dose of antibiotics. It did mean he qualified for a bed though, last night.

This was it then. September 12. My wedding day. It had been the longest walk over hot coals and broken bottles to get here. Now I prayed for, and believed I was owed, following winds for one day. I'd made so many bargains with every god and devil to get through today, that my soul was surely mortgaged a dozen times over. Anything from this day forward was a bonus.

At the end of this day I would have all I'd ever wanted and, though I still longed desperately to live, dying could never frighten me in the same way. Dave knocked on the door and poked his head in. "Morning," he said, awake on some level. "How're you feeling?" I hadn't got as far as figuring that out. I didn't feel as energised as I wanted, but I'd had three hours sleep, not to mention all the other stuff that was going on. "Okay. I think." I rubbed my eyes. "Let's go."

We stood outside the back entrance to the hospital, which was firmly locked. It was about a quarter to six, and the sign on the door informed us they wouldn't be unlocked before 6 a.m. A delivery driver was dropping off bread and pushed the buzzer to be let in. We asked nicely to sneak in behind him. "Security will come and let me in mate, but they'll tell you to go round the front. Sorry." The walk around to the front of the hospital, and then on to the ward which was just metres from where we'd started, was something like a quarter of a mile loop. Ordinarily, this wouldn't have been a problem of course, but I was suffering with the old ticker that morning. My heart kept kicking into fifth gear with little warning. A brisk walk was the opposite of what I needed. Still, we were on a pretty tight itinerary and had little chance but to head off round to the main entrance. I was breathing deeply, more in anticipation of my heart quickening than anything else. It occurred to me just how long it had been since I'd exerted myself. Months and months since I'd done more than a steady walk. Part of the

110

problem was that, during my lowest points in HDU, when I'd lapsed into unconsciousness, I'd been given adrenaline to bring me back. My heart rate, which was also elevated due to the infections it had been fighting off, had not yet returned to normal.

They were expecting us on the ward and had the antibiotics ready, but first were a quick set of observations, the standard temperature, blood pressure and heart rate tests. I'd settled on the bed but my heart chose this moment to turn over and double. I felt it go, and the turn sent a dizzying current to my brain. Immediately I was afraid. I didn't want any red flags causing alarm, for them or me. Still, the monitor went on and my heartbeat sounded out like a frantic symphony of beeps. The number even lit up in red and flashed for good measure. Dave's eyes widened. The nurse turned on her heels and walked out of the room. I was, with an imposed calmness, withdrawing into myself in concentration. In my mind I saw myself sitting cross-legged in a green clearing, surrounded by trees and crops of flowers. They were all swaying in a perfectly silent breeze, but I felt only the warming hum from the sun, a distant lamp. My breathing became very slow and I controlled every rising of my chest. Then I effingwell ordered my heart to slow down in a not very respectful way. When the nurse returned moments later, and accompanied by the sister on duty, my pulse had halved and was steadily falling. The hiccup was put down to the machine getting ahead of itself, which sometimes happened but, as I knew, had not on this occasion.

Antibiotics administered, we hot-footed it to the *Batmobile*, and then gunned it to the *Bat cave*, night staff wishing us good luck.

Back at home I got on with grilling some sausages and bacon for breakfast. My mind was elsewhere and I succeeded in cremating everything. But my guests dutifully chewed their way through it. While the others were free to begin getting ready at a leisurely pace, myself and best man Seb, the designated driver, had another trip to the hospital in store at around midday. Thankfully, that excursion went more smoothly and, when we got back, things were beginning to come together.

Sean had arrived with the buttonholes and having already figured out how the ties were fastened and where the pocket chain was supposed to go. He was busy passing on what he had learned to the others. Seb should jump in the shower first out of the two of us, we reasoned, he had hair. Meanwhile, until my turn, I had my suit out on the bed. I had lost even more weight since I'd had it fitted, and was prepared for it to hang off me.

I wondered how Mary was getting on at her Mum's. They had a real houseful; several relatives from Ireland and all nine bridesmaids. I tried to picture her, and thought what a different occasion today would have been had I not made it here. But here we were, for the grace of circumstance, the 50/50 rule. The toss of a coin.

Out of the shower, I put on the suit and looked in the mirror. I'd be lying if I said I was happy with how I looked. Gaunt, pale, bald. I sighed, feeling a pang of guilt for even going through with the wedding. I questioned whether it was fair to shackle myself to Mary, with what, for all I knew, could be a short period of ill-health followed by death. Was it right to do that to her? I chastised myself for thinking it. To walk away for the right reasons would actually be the cruellest thing I could do. So, I'd better get to the church then.

The Annunciation Catholic church in Chesterfield is fairly well hidden away, accessed by side road or footpath. When we got out of the car, I looked up at it, standing timelessly among the greys of the streets and the sky. This was the church at which Mary and I had attended Mass all those months ago. It was where I had closed my eyes and asked for something I thought was fair. I'd asked for enough time. I said a silent thank you for, in an hour-and-a-half, my wish would be granted.

Seb and Christian, the best men, grabbed me from either side for a photo, on which I felt sure my head would be glowing like a light bulb in the September air. But that would be the first of hundreds of photographs for which I'd have to pose that day. If all went to plan.

The photographer gathered the men together for a few shots on a patch of grass which was particularly badly pebble-dashed with dog poo, before we gave our shoes a good wipe and headed inside. People were arriving in a steady flow, and for the first time, I started to feel nervous about what was to come. There had been no time for a wedding rehearsal as seemed to be customary nowadays, and I realised I didn't really have the faintest idea what I was doing. I'd only been to a couple of weddings in my life and for one of those, my dad and Marion's no less, everyone had been dressed as cowboys, so I didn't know how much guidance I could take from that.

As if in answer to my doubts, Father McManus appeared and shook my hand welcomingly. A tall and stocky figure with a commanding voice, he cuts an imposing outline on the altar. But he is filled with such a depth and warmth that he immediately feels like a friend. Everything you could hope a priest to be I suppose. "How are you feeling, Richard?" Father McManus asked. "Okay thank you," I smiled. "I'm feeling well." "Don't worry about the ceremony today. I will guide you through it, so all you need to do is follow and you'll be fine. We've also put two chairs at the front so you can sit down through most of the service." I thanked him. The chairs were a good idea. I was uneasy about being on my feet for extended periods so I didn't know how the reception was going to pan out. I had this awful vision of me sitting in a chair for the whole evening shaking hands with a revolving queue of relatives and friends. I didn't want that. I would summon the strength from somewhere. That much I was sure of. It would hurt in the morning but today I was going to live every second.

Standing at the front of the church it seemed an age before I overheard that Mary was here. She was early, as I could have predicted. There's nothing of the diva about her. She was here to get married, not keep people waiting. I knew there would be a few photographs outside before the organ kicked in. I looked over my shoulder at my dad. He smiled. No prouder man has there ever been. Alongside him, Sean, Michael, Seb and Christian giggled about something amongst themselves. In that moment, all seemed right with the world. At long last, at the end of the longest night a dawn was breaking, and it was the most beautiful thing I'd ever felt.

The organ started. I straightened, eyes firmly fixed ahead. Father McManus caught my eye. "You're allowed to look, you know." Coming down the aisle, at a fair old speed it had to be said, was my Mary Ann, looking every inch a princess. I had not yet seen her dress, though she left a picture of it about the house. I knew what the folded square looked like from the outside, so would always return it to her, asking her not to be so careless with it. It was beautiful. She was beautiful, and, rather than feeling flooded by nerves or emotion, I felt suddenly very still and resolute. I had focussed on this day for so long. Now it was here I had settled into a determined mood. The calm of an athlete who has trained endlessly for one race. Like them, I expected I would hardly remember the race afterwards.

We held hands at the front of the church, in front of dozens of assembled family and friends; here to prove the proven, to tell everyone what they already knew. Father McManus welcomed everyone. "I often think," he began, "what shall I say at a wedding? Today I feel almost that I need not say anything. His words were very touching, and engaged, I think, with everyone in that place. I suppose our circumstances brought out the best in him, or gave him an opportunity at least to talk about what love really is. What it really means. If that sounds conceited, it isn't meant to. We both felt we couldn't love each other any more. As he promised, Father McManus led us through the ceremony, whispering when to "I will" and when to "I do." Mary must have asked me a dozen times during the service if I was okay. I was. I felt fine and, in any case, was too busy to notice otherwise. I checked my heartbeat a couple of times in true *Eric Morecambe* style. Once I found myself back in that clearing, where ghosts of a breeze lifted the leaves. I calmed myself again, letting all agitation bleed out of me.

"I now pronounce you, husband and wife," Father McManus said from nowhere. "You may kiss the bride." Someone cheered from the back, and ripples of applause pulled us into the moment and held us there. Right then I knew that we had won, whatever happened next.

Over the course of my treatment, I had come to see cancer as an opponent. It makes its moves and you make yours. As a being, it is malevolent and cruel, it serves no purpose, has nothing to gain. It plays by no rules, nor does it respect the boundaries of what you could term fairness. It only wants to kill and to deprive. I felt, as an entity and an enemy, it had fought to stop me reaching my wedding day, from getting married how and when we wanted. It craved that day, as if it hadn't taken enough already. But as the marriage was sealed with a kiss, we had defied cancer and that, I hoped, had wounded it in some small way.

Only when we reached the reception did it begin to rain, not that we could have cared less. We grabbed a handful of pictures outside and had the rest indoors. By the end of them I was flagging a bit and had to sit down for a minute. It was better to have a rest early on than risk burning out, I thought. Everyone had the chance to blow the froth off a couple before filing into the main hall via a "hallelujah handshake".

The food was exceptional, we thought, only Seb kept telling me throughout the meal how nervous he was about his speech. He produced a pen from somewhere and started making last minute revisions, which served to make me nervous about mine. My biggest fear was crumbling into an emotional wreck when I tried to speak. I was so happy and so grateful for the day turning out as it had so far, that I knew there was a risk that the emotion and the relief might get the better of me. I didn't think my speech was much cop either. I'd had time only to scribble a handful of sentences down on scrap paper. It could hardly be called polished. Still, Mary's dad had to go first, so that was something. It was his second father of the bride speech, and went down just as well as the first. He's a man of few words, so when he speaks you know he means it. He got huge applause. He sat.

This was it then. I hoped that, because today had been such a happy day, I wouldn't cry. It just wouldn't fit. I stood up and greeted everyone. Then said: "You wonder what you're going to do with your hair on your wedding day, don't you?" It was the best I could come up with to just get the obvious out of the way. They seemed to like it. The speech went well, and I thanked Mary for picking me up every day through good, bad and worse. I said she is a miracle and that, today, I was marrying my guardian angel. Emma's Dave and Michael had already colluded to try and start a standing ovation after my speech 'no matter how crap it is.' So, as I sat down, I was passed by everyone going the other way. It's a strange feeling, having an ovation, an outpouring of good wishes to you. You suddenly feel validated.

Seb and Christian's speeches were both great in their different styles, packed with gags and tales of drunken revelry. I felt proud of the two of them, though I wasn't sure from which part of my character. They just felt like good friends I supposed.

Things were packed away for the disco and people passed the time with a beer or two. I knew I would not be drinking much that I wouldn't want to but had asked Dr. Cowdrey if I was allowed to drink. "Oh yes," he said. "Get well tanked!" My favourite piece of advice from a healthcare professional ever. Once the first dance was over, which both of us were dreading, the evening could be a little more relaxing for us. The time was sailing by as everyone said it would. But the day had blossomed into this beautiful bubble. Everyone there was enjoying themselves so much and there was a sea of love in the room, splashing up the walls. All the time I'd been in hospital and thought about the wedding, I had this vision of Mary and I on the dance floor, swinging each other about to the Libertines' song *Don't look back into the Sun*. It's really fast and one of my favourites. When the song came on, it was even more magical. *"Don't look back into the sun/Don't you know that your time has come/And they never thought it'd come for you."*

Saturday September 13 2008. Course 4: Day 33.

Twas the morning after the night before and I was moving like a marionette. From some dark recess I had summoned strength enough to still be standing, with occasional dancing, until about 4 a.m. I was paying for every minute but what a night. I had the biggest smile on my face that nothing was going to shift, not even a 6 a.m. alarm sounding.

I left my lady wife sleeping soundly as I slipped out of the door in jeans and a jacket. My dad was waiting in the corridor. I think he's better at getting up than me. He put an arm around me. "How does it feel?" That was really a bigger question than he realised. How did it feel to be married? How did it feel to have stuck two fingers up at cancer and made it through the day? How did I feel now it was over? "It feels good," I told him. "Sleepy but good."

The pattern of that day set the standard for the next few, as far as timescales and travel were concerned. We arrived at hospital early for my dose of antibiotics, left knowing I would be back after lunchtime before having one more, 'the nightcap' I called it, sometime around midnight. It was quite a punishing routine, it soon became clear. Back at the hotel, bed was all I could think about. I don't think Mary's ever looked so pleased to see me as when I got there. Sleep.

We woke and opened a few wedding cards. Perhaps it was because of the circumstances of our wedding or maybe we were just splendid people, but donations were very generous indeed. We decided to have a fancy holiday, something neither of us had done before. As there was much needed to spend money on in the house, we had wanted to save something, but we'd never earned enough to do before. We had a cooked breakfast in the hotel and the rest of the day was just a leisurely foray into what this married lark was all about.

At this point, the rest of Richard's journal changes, as it is written in free-flow form as opposed to under calendar dates.

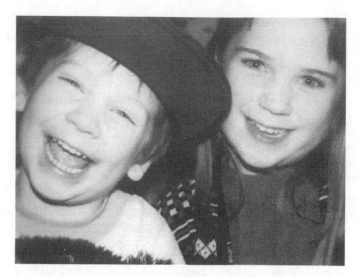

"Carefree days with sister Emma"

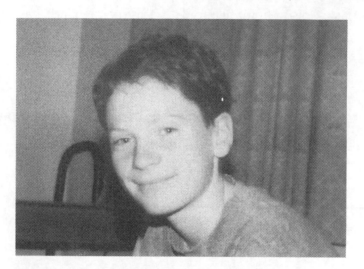

"Handsome beyond words"

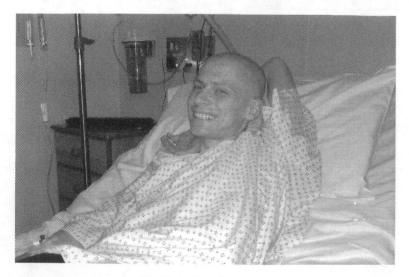

"Still smiling"

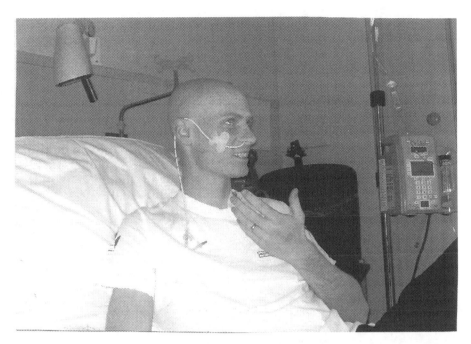

"Ever the story teller"

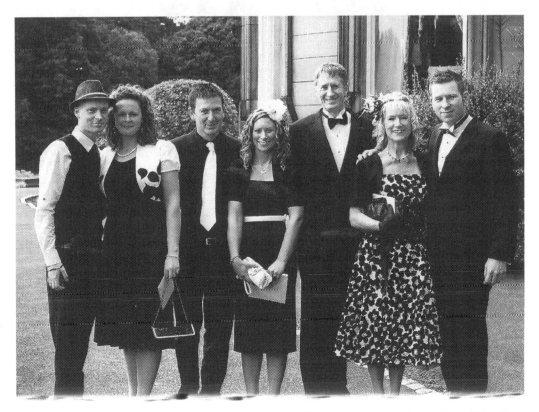

"With Mary, Dave, Emma, Dad, Marion and the Groom at Ben's Wedding"

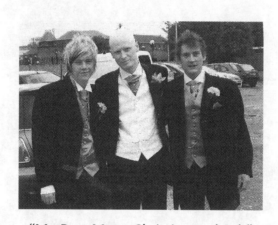

"My Best Men - Christian and Seb"

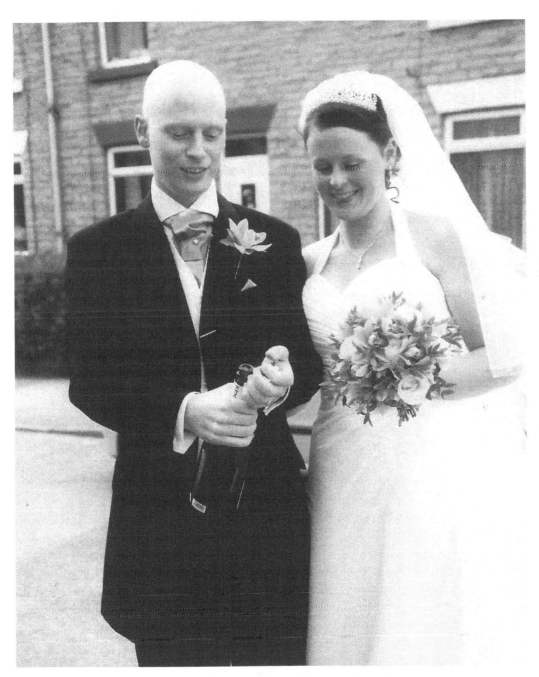

"What a celebration - We got there"

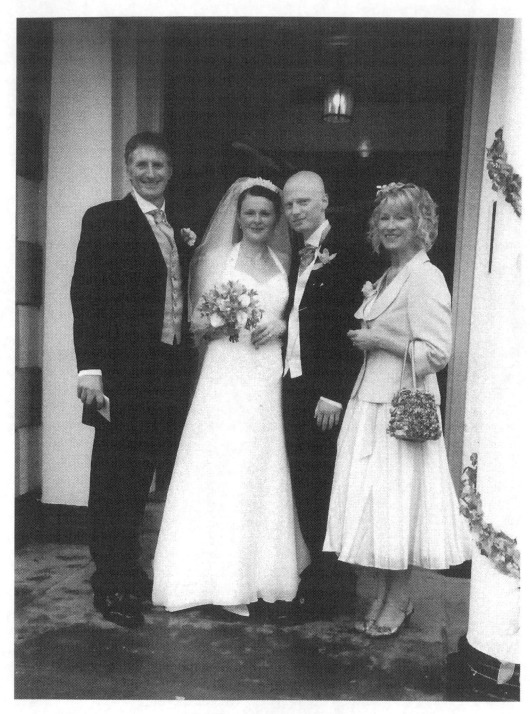

"With Dad and Marion"

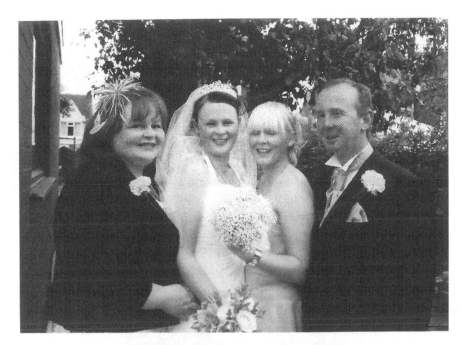

"Mary with her Mum, sister Helen and Dad"

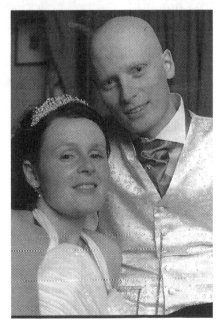

" A dream come true"

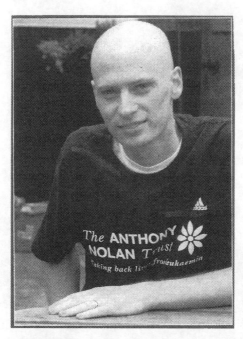

"Press photo - preparing for the London Marathon"

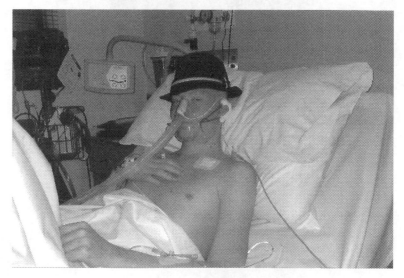

"In the wars, but still got style"

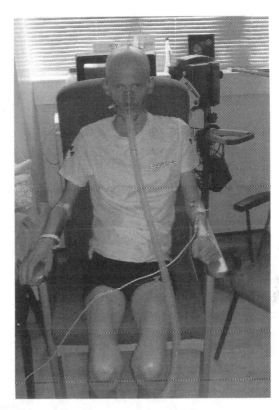

"At the end of Course 6, fighting to come home"

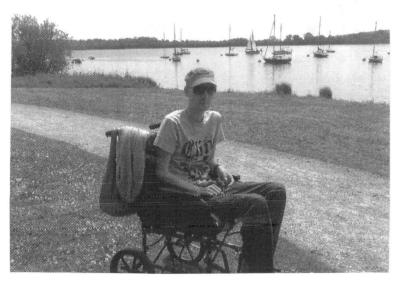

"Carsington Water, after Course 6"

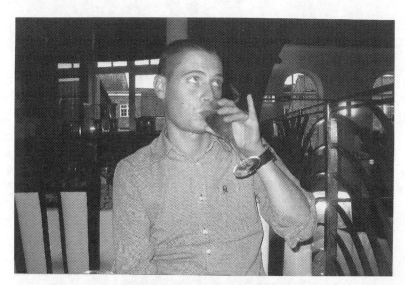

"White wine with yet more class!"

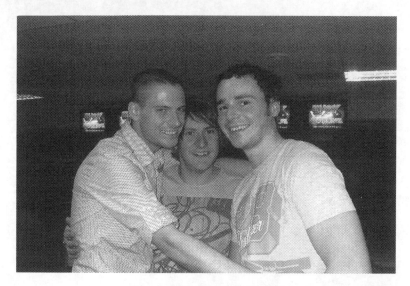

"With Seb and Michael"

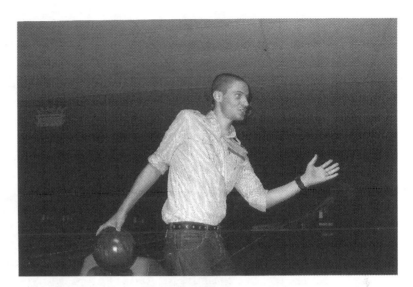

"Stylishly facing the wrong way"

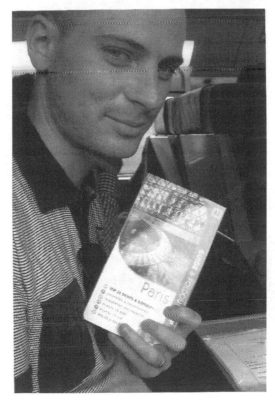

"Unauthorised trip to Paris"

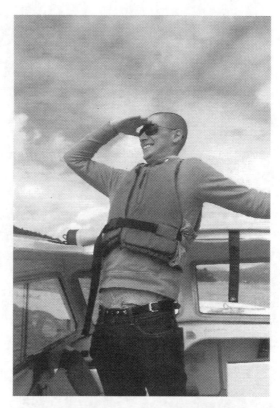

"Ahoy there in Bowness"

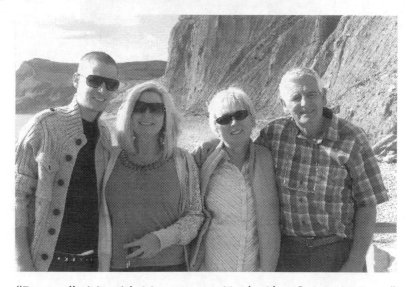

"Farewell visit with Mum to see Uncle Alan & Auntie Anna"

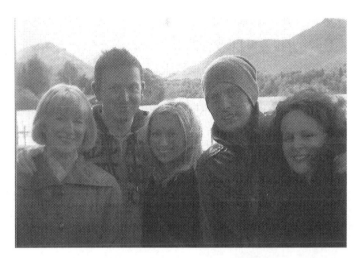

"Last family holiday in the Lakes"

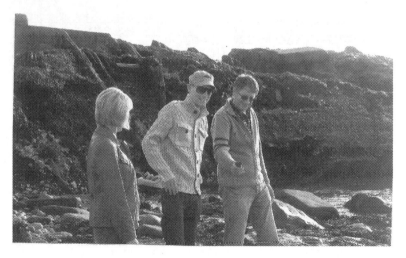

"Skimming stones with Dad and Marion"

Next Steps to Recovery

September 2008

Mary and I stole away to Manchester for a couple of nights in a hotel. Aside from my baldness there was nothing to distinguish us from the other couples huddled at the platform edge. We spent the day having nice meals and shopping. I bought Mary a leather jacket; hardly redress. It was a lovely few days.

When we got back we just took everything very slowly. We didn't make too many plans to overburden ourselves, but nor did we just vegetate. I kept moving, and felt stronger day by day. The next thing on the horizon was the stem cell harvest, which the doctors had agreed to let me do post-chemo, rather than in between courses which is customary. I still had my Hickman line in for this purpose, as it was a good way for them to get at my blood. I couldn't wait to get rid of the thing – the final reminder of where I'd been. In order to keep the line flowing, I was going in once a week, on a Wednesday, to have it flushed at clinic in Chesterfield.

October 2008

Unfortunately I soon started noticing I felt unwell every Wednesday evening. This only really pointed to one thing. We had a routine appointment with the transplant nurse, Andrea, in Sheffield that day and she took some cultures from my line before I left.

The following day, while we were out Christmas shopping, Andrea phoned me back. She sounded really pained to tell me that a bug was growing in the line. Every time it was flushed, it just sent more of the toxins into my blood. It needed to come out. I was disappointed but quickly resigned myself with the comfort of knowing the line had to go anyway. An appointment had already been made at Chesterfield to remove the line, which I would have done as an outpatient.

Something about the procedure unnerved me, so I repeatedly played it out going well in my head. How would it feel to be without it again? Strange, I was sure. Eventually Dr. Woodward joined us in the room with a small instrument tray. We talked for a minute about what was to come then I peeled off my shirt. Dr. Woodward got to work putting in painkilling injections and talking himself through every step of what he did. Mary was asked to leave, so she kissed me and headed off to the canteen. What happened next I will remember for as long as I live.

The way they remove lines at Chesterfield is make a little cut into the hole from which the catheter hangs. This is to release the cuff, a small spongy piece of material designed to bolt the line in place. After that, with varying degrees of coercion, the line should slide out like a piece of spaghetti. That's the theory.

What happened in my case though, is this. Dr. Woodward made his incision. "Okay," he said, "and now we should just be able to ... "He gripped the line as though it was something between a great snake and the finest chain necklace. He pulled, then a little harder and my Hickman line snapped. Dr. Woodward, the nurse who was assisting and I all just stared at it hanging there from his hand, bloody and incomplete. "That's never happened to me before," Dr. Woodward said. "It's never happened to me either," I said, feeling my heart turn over. "I need a scalpel and tweezers to see if I can get a grip on what's left." He dashed out of the room, a little flustered. The nurse and I both kind of awkwardly existed there, locked in the unexpectedness of it all.

Mary soon got wind something had gone wrong. She ran into a colleague in the canteen who asked how I was getting along with things. Mary said, "Dr. Woodward is taking his Hickman line out." Mary said her friend's eyes widened before she confessed to have just left another ward where Dr. Woodward was pacing around asking for tweezers and/or a surgeon. Mary's heart dropped. She said she remembered thinking, "Why can't even the smallest thing go right?"

Back on the ward she savaged Dr. Woodward, but to be fair to the man I don't believe any of what happened was his fault. What had happened was that the internal scar tissue around my line had healed so well there was no way it was coming out for anyone. I wondered if there had been extra scar tissue because of the clumsy way the line went in, during which I felt every millimetre of its endeavour into my artery. The long and the short of it, though, was: "so now what we gonna do?" Theatre was booked out, I kept hearing people say. Then I'd always seem to overhear the word 'lancings,' which conjured an unpalatable image. I don't know why, but when someone says theatre, the other person must fit the word 'lancings' into their next sentence. I think it's a surgeons' game that goes over my head, though I too found myself joining in. Someone would phone me up: "Hey, you having your op today?" "No," I'd grumble, "theatre's booked up - lancings." I also heard there was a particularly bad dog bite case. All in all it was about two full days in hospital before they called me down to theatre, having cleared all the lancings, and what was left of my Hickman line was removed surgically. It's why on my chest I have a five inch scar.

Trauma aside, the line was out and I could get back on with whatever it was I'd been doing before all this. There was a very real sense, all the time that I wanted to do more, achieve more. Although simple things pleased me more than ever, I seemed to thirst after things to do. On documentaries, when a witness is being interviewed, it may flash up their name and then the word 'Survivor' – Auschwitz, Titanic, whatever. That's what I was now, a survivor, and I felt the duties of my new role were distinct. I had to gather as much love, joy and experience together as humanly possible to do in a lifetime. Now, you might ask, isn't that what we're all trying to do anyway? I'd agree, but think we're too distracted by that HD plasma screen. Walking hand in hand with being a survivor was survivor's guilt. I'd made it this far for reasons none of us understood. Many more had not understood this, in time. They were all real people with real families who played cricket on a Sunday and shooed flies from their sandwiches afterwards. Their stories didn't get endings. Not real ones. They just stopped writing. So, why them and not me? To an extent, it doesn't matter. The way it helps me to think of it, is this, my death wouldn't have benefited anyone else. Nobody would have 'got my place' had I left. I simply do not believe it works like that. Guilt is such a heavy thing to carry, particularly if it's misplaced. So I learned to put it down.

November 2008

As a lead up to the stem cell harvest, I needed to have four day's worth of GCSF injections, which stimulate the bone marrow. The idea is that your body produces so many of these stem cells, that is, ones which can become whatever cell is needed, that they spill over into the blood stream. From there, they can be skimmed off by a machine with two ports, blood in and blood out. The upside was it sounded favourable to a general anaesthetic and the cells being taken en mass from my bone marrow. The down side was spending four to five hours rigged up to the machine and not being allowed to move your arm. Oh, and sometimes it took up to three days instead of one. The doctors had a yield of cells in mind, and at the end of the day the number harvested were counted. Presumably with a microscope and a pinhead. They needed in the region of 2.5 million. Judging the GCSF is a tricky thing. Your stem cell production will reach a certain peak and, with any luck, that will be the day you do your harvest. A person might be sent away until the next day because their stem cells have not fully mobilised, or there's the other possibility: you've peaked and it was yesterday.

We went in for a morning blood test to see if I had enough stem cells in my blood to attempt the procedure. This would be an indication, to my mind at least, of how well my bone marrow was functioning. Normally, people do the stem cell harvest after the second or third chemo, when their marrow has not been so assaulted. Many people, even when doing this earlier, can't mobilise enough stem cells to make it viable.

A charming Asian doctor, all smiles and wisdom, leaned around the door frame, "You're ready," she said. I'd allowed my mind to run away with me a bit about this. I'd read the cover notes and there was talk of finding veins in groins and necks when suitable ones in the arms could not be found. I also imagined we'd be talking about a pretty big needle, which I was right about. But the ladies who worked there really knew their stuff and have big hearts, so they soon put me at ease. Once on the machine, it was simply a matter of staying pretty much as still as possible, within reason, mainly the right arm as this housed the needle. Because the needle was so long, bending the arm would have torn me, and caused a weird and wonderful new set of problems. This led to the faintly hilarious situation where Mary had to turn the pages of my magazine for me and feed me flapjack. At one stage, one of the nurses asked if I would like the radio on. I thought it could be a distraction. "Yes, please," I said. She pressed a button on it and the faintest, most inaudible sound came out. She walked away to do something else and I remember thinking, "C'mon. Dogs can't even hear that!" If it was a digital stereo it would have been volume 1, a number which only exists so you can crank it to at least eight. I couldn't even tell if it was music or discussion. I could just hear something, like a fly buzzing very far away. But it did make us chuckle so that's points in the bag as far as I'm concerned.

I think I did an extra half an hour or so on the machine to make sure they didn't come up just short, which would have been annoying. But there was still a very good chance I would be back tomorrow. We gathered our things and headed out into dropping temperatures, the air dry and cold. Later that evening, I was telephoned by Mandy, one of the nurses from the harvest clinic. She told me they had gathered about 1.6 of the 2.5m they needed to harvest, a figure which, she said was disappointing given the stem cell levels in my blood were quite good. On day 2 they would need to get 0.9m out of me when my levels will have been tailing off after the injections. I could see it being a longer day than had gone before. We went to bed at a sensible hour with the intention of getting there in good time.

Now, if you had an appointment for a potentially life enhancing procedure, at great cost to the NHS, you'd probably take care to keep it wouldn't you? I, however, managed to turn up almost an hour-and-a-half late. What happened was, and I feel eternally embarrassed about this, was complete traffic gridlock. It had snowed in places and everyone in Sheffield had simultaneously forgotten how to drive, like some comet had hit the motoring gene. I was getting more and more embarrassed as I watched my appointment time approach and slide by, waving, while we hunched over in a metal box hardly moving. I ended up jumping out and power-walking the last quarter mile. They understood. It was okay. But we pressed on. They hooked me back up again and I stayed on for about five-and-a-half hours. It was tougher the second day. My back and arm were already aching before I started. Later on we got the call. "We got enough. 2.5m exactly."

It was around this time that I first heard about Rita Strong. Dr. Strong was one of the haematology consultants at Chesterfield. She had given me my diagnosis and I have nothing but the greatest of respect not only for how she did that, but, I think, every subsequent clinical decision she made in my care. I had, of course, noticed she had been away from the hospital for a while. At first I thought it may have been a long holiday, or bereavement. But decided it was most probably illness, due to the length of time that had elapsed. I thought it impolite to ask. Drs. Cowdrey and Woodward had picked up the slack and were keeping Durrant Ward and the clinics going, but I got a sense they must be up against it.

As it turned out, Dr. Strong had breast cancer. She was being treated at Weston Park in Sheffield and doing well by all accounts. You had to pity her doctor I suppose. I'd always admired Dr. Strong. Fiercely intelligent, but she had a true doctor's heart. I suspect too many go into medicine motivated by ego and status. Not her. I'd heard from more than one member of staff at Chesterfield that she and Dr. Cowdrey were the best two doctors in the place. I couldn't say, that's just what I heard. But the news of Dr. Strong seemed to sit like a splinter in my chest and, for a day or two; she was all I could think about. The thought I couldn't get beyond was that Dr. Strong had done so much in her career to snatch back lives from cancer, and so much to improve the quality of life of those living with it. Now it wanted her. Viewing cancer as an element, as I did, I couldn't help but wonder if it had come-a-knocking. She is known to cancer. What scared me was, how much does it want her? There are so many types of the disease its mind-bending and they can vary in aggression. I suppose the bottom line is, if it really wants you there's nothing you can do. It's a three line whip. If it spreads to your organs and bones quickly you don't really have a move. Two patients with the same diagnosis and prognosis, may have the same treatment and yet one may live, one may die. But you have to consider the complications of the treatment, which can be as deadly as the disease itself. I suppose one of the hardest things was that, when I was ill, Dr. Strong helped me. Now she was ill and I could do nothing at all.

The London Marathon

It was one afternoon at home, after I'd breathlessly returned from walking to the shop, that I decided I should run the London Marathon. Mary was back at work now and I'd often find myself sitting on the sofa, thinking about things. Such a shocking and life-changing set of events had just befallen me and now I wasn't sure what to do. I felt like a fish, pulled from the sea to be poked and prodded before being tossed back in. I was still kind of floundering around the boat, unsure what the ocean held for me anymore. I don't know what triggered the thought on that day. Nothing that I recall, but I was conscious that, for some time, I had been searching for something. Something to work towards, to build. A goal. Seb and Helen were already signed up for the marathon and I remember feeling a pang of jealousy when I heard. Running the London Marathon has always been an ambition of mine. I loved to run and have the right build for it. At school I was in the cross country team, but was never one of the outstanding runners. I think I was making up numbers but I enjoyed it. Getting out there in the muck and the cold. That's living. But this was a big step. It was December, the race was in April. Was that enough time for someone in my condition to prepare? After all, not long had passed since I was in HDU unable to walk. Was it even safe for me to take part? But the lure of it was too great. I checked the dates and saw the run would take place almost exactly a year from when I was diagnosed. If I finished it, that would be a real achievement. It would not be completing a marathon 12 months after finishing treatment, but a year from finding out. I had something to prove to myself. I wanted to take back control of my body, which had baffled and disappointed me so much in the preceding months. But I also wanted to provide hope for people like me, earlier in the timeline of their treatment, who didn't think they would ever feel normal again. Then there was the part of me that just wanted to do it as a 'fuck you' to cancer. Even if it got me in the end, I wanted it to know it had been in a fight.

I didn't know if there would even be places left in the marathon at this late stage. A quick check of the website told me all the individual places had been assigned already, by ballot, but charities themselves still had places. I scanned the charities with 'golden bonds' as they call them, leukaemia care, children with leukaemia, Marie Curie. Who to choose? It would be them who ultimately chose me, I reasoned, so I should probably apply to a handful. I filled out several forms on line for cancer charities. I wanted to run for one of them but would run for anyone ultimately. I clicked on the Anthony Nolan Trust banner to see if they still had places. That charity, which administrates the bone marrow register, was my first choice. "All our places for the London Marathon have now been filled, but we do have spaces remaining for the New York Marathon, Tokyo Marathon ..." I felt a bit deflated. Had I left it too late? As soon as I had the idea in my head a very big boulder had started rolling. I can be quite singular of mind when I need to be. Something made me fill out a form anyway and I posted it off.

When Mary came home from work I had my serious face on, which is similar to my 'been-up-to-something' face, which of course, I had. "What's going on?" Mary said, key frozen in the door. "Has something happened?" "No, no," I said, "no, no, nothing can be said to have happened." "So why are you being weird? Have you bought me a present?" It tickles me that whenever I act slightly out of character, or make a bang in the back bedroom, Mary's first instinct is always that I have bought her a present. "No," I laughed, "sorry." Then I chanced: "It's better than that." Now she was really intrigued. I sighed, not knowing how she was going to react to my proposal. I guessed her first instinct would be to protect me and that she may say it was a bad idea. "Okay," I began, "well, you know we've talked about me having goals? It being important to work towards things.""Yes," she replied, impatiently. "Well I'd like to run the London Marathon. In April. If I can get a place." I scanned Mary's face and it tightened a little, as though I'd just said something hurtful. She thought about it for a moment. "I just want you to be safe. I think you might be trying to do too much too soon. I don't know if you're well enough yet." God bless her. It was a softer answer than I had expected, as, the more I thought about the idea, the more I was questioning it. But the way I saw it, I had believed in myself, trained myself, deprived myself and stretched myself through this ordeal and I could do the same now. People always say a marathon is the hardest thing they've ever done. After my year, a marathon would be hot butter. Through all my treatment I had the belief that I would get better, that if the odds were against me I would beat them. I had the same belief that I could run this marathon. I just wasn't able to run anywhere just yet. Anyway, I didn't even have a place yet so there was no point getting ahead of myself. Mary and I talked for a while and she soon came round and gave me full support. I think she recognised that I needed this.

I'd already received a few rejection notices when I got the call. I absent-mindedly pinned the phone to my ear with my shoulder. "Hello Richard, I'm calling from the Anthony Nolan Trust. Is now a good time?" I was peeling parsnips. "Er yes, now's ..... great," I said, taking the phone in my hand. We ran through a few pleasantries and then she started asking me questions, including what shirt size I was. My heart started beating faster. Did this mean I had a place? The girl's voice on the other end, all cute and childlike, told me they'd be happy to have me on the team. I silently struck a pose, and felt as though I'd just been filled to the top with life. "Really? Thank you," I said. "You've made my week." I felt incredibly thankful. Here I was, signing myself up to an agonisingly painful tour of the capital and pledging to raise £1,500. But it felt like a gift. I stayed on the phone another few minutes, during which we thanked each other gratuitously. I put down the phone and did the only thing that felt right. A little dance. "We're going to Wem-ber-ley" was echoing in my head. Though that wasn't strictly true, the sentiments of the chant were perfect. A big event was coming and I was going to be there. This was just what I needed. My recovery had been good but it had been rudderless. Now I had the drive to bounce back and be even stronger than before.

When Mary came in from work and I told her, she said, "You'd better tell your Dad and Marion." Their reaction was fairly typical of immediate family. They said no. By what authority was unclear, but they were saying no. My dad cupped his ears, "You can't. There's no way you'll be fit enough." I explained to them that my first few training runs had gone quite well, and I could already run for half-an-hour or more. That would have been nothing to me a couple of years earlier but I was starting from zero. Each run had been longer and felt easier. I was just testing the water really, checking the damage. My Mum was similarly horrified; convinced that over-exerting myself could bring back the leukaemia. But everyone came around quite quickly when they realised I was determined about it. Now I couldn't wait to get stuck into some training.

There's nothing quite like running for me. Solitary and honest. I don't like treadmills. Why coop yourself up watching MTV when there are a million miles of streets waiting to be pounded. Go out and beat a hill; sprint the block faster than you did last week. Being outdoors is the very essence of that freedom. I knew the value of my legs now, and I was sure I could reignite my passion for running. I ran later that day, just an easy few miles, and smiled at the fact that, for a split second on every step, I was flying.

Alternative Therapy

I had never been one for alternative therapies. Science had done me proud so far thank you. But sometimes in life you think 'What's the harm?' They were my thoughts when it was suggested I visit a healer. A man with 'recognised' healing powers was holding a session at a church in Alfreton, near to where Mary's mum lived. It was free to see him. I couldn't conscience the idea of the leukaemia coming back so I was willing to try, if not anything, something from left field. I, quite embarrassingly, turned up an hour late. Again. This was due to a third party telling us the wrong time. But, after a light telling-off from a nun, Mary and I sat down in the pews at the back. We immediately spotted Janice, a friend of Mary's family. Despite being diagnosed with MS many years ago, Janice had defied doctors' expectations by exhibiting very few symptoms over the years. This she put down to a regime of treatments, therapies and anything else she read about that may help prevent onset. She's a very kind and gentle lady. We smiled at her and she looked happy and hopeful. I felt a little apprehensive about what was to come, and couldn't look far away from the heavy oak door at the front of the church. People around us were praying, or sitting silently, gazing towards the front.

The decor in the church was sparse, twelve figurines adorned the pillars, depicting Jesus' journey carrying the cross. The door at the front opened and a woman came out in a long black coat. The first thing I noticed was that she was crying. Very freely, unashamedly. My stomach stirred as the woman chose a seat at the front and sort of fell into it. Then she went very still. A nun consoled her, before coming towards me to tell me it was my turn. Mary turned to Janice, "Would you like to go first? You were here before us." Janice took up the offer as I think she had somewhere to go. The oak door closed behind her, keeping its secrets. I scanned the walls looking for blemishes, but they were perfect. I wondered why I was looking for something wrong or broken. I'm a very sceptical person and I wasn't quite sure why I was here. Maybe miracles can only happen within well-plastered walls.

I'd become a grand-master in wasting time. Hospital teaches you to set your expectations so low your thoughts become a soothing drone. It's a bit like meditation without the leg-ache. I withdrew into myself for the hour Janice was in that room, while Mary, who does not wait well, fidgeted and checked her watch. Eventually Janice emerged and I saw that her face was streaked with tears. She nodded a goodbye as she passed us, but she was really crying hard. What had I signed up for? I felt emotionally fragile at that time. I was still rebuilding all aspects of myself. I hadn't come here to cry myself silly. I could do that in my own time.

We were led to the front and through the oak door to a little room with four chairs laid out in a square. An Irish woman greeted us, while I could hear a man clinking a teaspoon on china in a little tea room to my right. He stepped into the room and it was immediately apparent that he was a priest, either that or on his way to a saints and sinners party. He too had an Irish twang. We were invited to sit and the two of them began asking me questions about the nature of my illness. Then the question I was fearing; "What is your faith?" My eyes went upwards and I paused. "I'm open to beliefs," I said. The Irish lady smiled and put a hand on my knee. "Don't worry. We have enough faith for everyone here." She whispered something to the Father and then said; "Now, Richard, we've been doing these sessions a long time and what we've discovered is that when people become very unwell, it is a result of something traumatic from their past, something they haven't dealt with properly, becoming manifest in cancers and such like."

Already, she was losing me. Mentally I was stepping backwards out of the room. But I'm not so pompous as to believe I know everything, and I had promised I would surrender to this. Even if it made me feel a right prune. "Tell me, Richard," she went on, "did something bad happen to you a couple of years ago, because that's when it will have been, experience tells us. Do you have any painful memories of that time?" My eyebrows flattened and I thought about it. Two or three years ago I had been having the time of my life. Mary and I went out about three times a week, along with Seb, before he got together with Helen. The only thing traumatic was the hangovers. "That was actually a pretty fun period in my life," I said, a little embarrassed. I was young, care-free, in love. "Did you lose anyone close to you?" the woman asked, which kind of snapped me out of a highlights memory-montage I was enjoying. "No," I said, trying not to sound cagey. They changed tack.

"Mary, is there anything you can think of?" I could sense her uneasiness, even though, as instructed, I had my eyes closed. "Well, the only bad thing to happen in his life before this was his parents splitting up." The pair of them made a sound as though they'd just caught sight of the animal they were tailing. They had their 'in'. The reason I didn't mention my parents' divorce was because it was so long ago. I was 10. That didn't seem to matter. "Richard," the woman said, for it was she who did most of the talking, "it maybe that your parents' separating and the effect that had on you caused your leukaemia." I bristled, and my legs very nearly carried me out of there on their own. I swallowed a cube of anger that dug its corners into my throat. She was talking again. "Tell us what happened." What's to explain? I told her in no uncertain terms: "It was a painful time in my life but it was a long time ago and I have dealt with it, moved on. I have a good relationship with both my parents, feel no bitterness towards either of them and recognise they were ill-suited. The end."

Quite succinct, I thought. "Well," she said, "it is our belief that you haven't actually dealt with it, despite what you say." This woman was making detailed psycho-analytical suppositions about me when she didn't know me from *Bruce Forsythe*. I tightened. I wasn't there any more. Not really. "Please tell us your memories of the time. Were there arguments? Did you feel pulled in two directions?" "There's not much to say really. They had differences for years, probably brought out the worst in each other, so they decided to split." "Was anyone else involved?" I shifted in my seat, "Yes," I said. "On whose side?" "My Mum's." "I see. And was it painful for you to find out about this other person? How did you find out?" I knew she was going to have a field day with this. "Well, obviously, my sister and I knew nothing of this other person. When it all came out my Mum sat the two of us down in a *McDonald's* and told us they were divorcing." "In a *McDonalds*?" I coughed, "Yes." "And how did you feel about having to deal with something so private in such a public place?" "It wasn't ideal." "Richard, I want you to imagine you are back in that *McDonalds* with your sister and your mother is telling you that she and your dad are separating. Go back to that moment." I remembered. Sticky red gloss decor. Smell of fries and disinfectant. Feet zipping by on the pavement outside. A corner booth. "Now I want you to imagine that, just after being told, you see Jesus coming into *McDonalds*." I hear he is more of *a KFC* man, but I didn't say so. "What does Jesus say to you?" I delve back into my memory and look at the door and, sure enough, in comes Jesus. He doesn't walk, more glide along the floor. I don't tell them that in my vision he is wearing a top hat. He stands there, unsmiling, looking at me. "Now what does Jesus say to you?" I look at Jesus, he looks back. No words are exchanged. "I can't see him saying anything," I said. "What would you want him to say?" I think about this for some time as I watch the light glint off Jesus' top hat.

They're trying their best to make me cry, I thought, to illicit an emotional outpouring so that I feel purged. Healed. But I've cried my tears for that time in my life. It's long passed. "Just some reassurance," I suggested. I got a sense that I wasn't playing ball as they'd like me to. "Now," the woman said, "did you feel angry with your mother at the time?" "A little, probably, but not anymore. Not at all." "I want you to imagine shaking her." "Shaking her?" "Taking her by the shoulders and shaking her, telling her that she hurt you." I smothered a laugh. "I don't want to do that." It didn't seem very Christian to me to be recommending it. There's no commandment that reads: Thou shalt not shake, but I thought, on the whole, it went against the charitable spirit of the faith. "There's nothing wrong with imagining it. Doing so may help you."

I went quiet for a minute, giving them time to believe I was attacking my mother in some *Norman Bates* fashion. I wasn't. I love my Mum. We're past it. "Now," she said, presumably after she thought my Mum had been suitably thrashed. "Where was your father when this was happening, when you were in *McDonalds*?" I didn't know the answer. *Burger King*? "I think he was at home, waiting for us." "Did you feel angry that he wasn't there?" Eyes still closed, "No." "But would you have preferred him to be there with you?" A leading question. "Yes." "There are obviously some feelings buried deep within you, feelings of anger and disappointment in how your parents acted. What I want you to do is picture them both in front of you. Tell them that they hurt you. Then tell them you want to forgive them, but you don't yet. You can choose when you are ready to forgive."

Okay, I thought. Now! I was ready for this to end. They asked me to stand, before they began laying their hands on me and chanting under their breath. "Amen, Lord," he said, and it was over. I opened my eyes, blinking under the spotlights. "How do you feel?" she asked me. I tried to think of a diplomatic answer, given that I felt no different to when I'd walked in. "Good," I settled on. The two of them hugged the two of us. We were wished the very best of luck and God's love, then we parted company. Outside, in the car, Mary stopped me, "I'm so sorry," she said. "I just wanted to pick you up and carry you out of there. The things they were saying just aren't you or what you're about." I tossed her a smile, "It was an experience." Let's go home.

Christmas 2008 and the New Year

Christmas was beginning to loom. I successfully ignored it for months though its imagery was everywhere. Mary's Auntie Sheila, a formidable fundraiser, had the idea to raise some cash for Durrant Ward's staff Christmas party. That sounded a great idea to Mary and me, so we volunteered to do whatever we could to help. The format was a handbag and jewellery party at Sheila's featuring the creations of her friend Sonya, who made bags, jewellery and ornaments herself, as well as retailing other pieces. Mary baked a cake and I took charge of the raffle, which would be where the cash was gathered. The day went really well and we raised the best part of £200. Mary and I had a think about it and decided giving staff cash for a night out would be too complicated, the hospital had forms which had to be completed and then they would have to divide it somehow. And what about those who couldn't go? No, there was another way. We went to the supermarket and bought a trolley-full of wine. A trolley-full. It was wonderful. Red, white, rosé. A good mixture. We needed two wheelchairs to deliver it all, bags hanging from every handle and hook, clunking down the ward. It was nice to do some small thing for the staff and their families. God knows they deserved a lot more.

Christmas turned into quite a lavish affair, inevitably. I mean, why hold back? We threw ourselves into it and spent far too much on one another. Money had never really meant much to either of us before, now it meant very little indeed. In fact, all of life's minutia had faded into the background where they belonged. That's the beauty of near death experiences; they're very effective at illuminating what is important and what is not. We had a lovely Christmas Day at Mary's mum's, and in the evening I got monumentally drunk with Seb and Michael. That was the first time I'd been properly drunk in eight months.

On Boxing Day, my dad and Marion came round and I cooked two enormous curries. I love making a mess in the kitchen.

New Year was spent in Derby with some of our friends. We were conscious that time seemed to be ghosting past at real speed. We were keeping busy but life was accelerating all around us, sucking us back into the rat race. I was determined not to put any of what had happened behind me. I'd had a traumatic but ultimately positive learning experience. I think the brain naturally tries to forget painful memories. But I didn't want that to happen to me. I was using them. It just took a little thought every day, a little reminder that I was not the person I was before. My life was not what it was. I felt like I'd been given a valuable tool, like I knew something most people didn't know.

January 2009

Fast approaching was the date of my two-monthly blood test and then, the following day, I was going back to work. I was nervous about both, but also excited. Both had the power to validate my health. I felt sure they would. I was running further and further and feeling better than ever, stronger, hungrier. When the blood test came, the results were all normal, other than a low platelet count. Dr. Woodward assured me this was common for this stage. "How would you feel about me running the London Marathon then," I dropped in. I will never forget his response, "Good Lord!" I took that as a full blessing. I'd have done it anyway.

My nervousness about going back to work centred on two things. Firstly, I didn't want a fuss. If I'd have walked in the door and been greeted by a banner it would have made me uncomfortable. The second concern was that I had been doing the job I was returning to only a matter of weeks. Would I remember what I was doing? But, as with so much in my life at that time, I shrugged it off. What did it really matter? If they made a fuss, let them. If I was thrown in at the deep end, I'd swim. In the end, I should have given my colleagues more credit. They were superb and made me feel welcome instantly. No fuss. I felt a weight of gratitude to my employer, Johnston Press, who had really gone both guns to help me when I was off. I was contracted for four months' full pay when sick. They paid me for eight. The value of that was more than the money it equated to. One of the first things I did when I got back was email the Managing Director to say thank you. I had more than 1,000 emails waiting for me. I just deleted them all. I love my job. Life was a splendid thing. Every second sang with possibilities, glowed with the warmth of simply being. Maybe it was too good to last.

I was now seriously fit. Give me my iPod, my new trainers, open the door and stand back. I could run for two hours plus pretty easily. Up and down hills, dodging cars, down backstreets, main roads and rarely-trodden footpaths, rain, ice. I loved them all, especially a long punishing hill. My lungs felt like gallon drums, my legs like trees. My heartbeat, at rest, had slowed to an occasional whump. It felt glorious. A limitless freedom. It was like passing your driving test and the world suddenly feeling so much smaller, more accessible. Only I didn't need a car.

Every time I thought about the marathon the hair on my neck would stand on end. Other than to get married, I had never wanted anything more. In fact, I was already getting ahead of myself. I was thinking "When's the New York Marathon? When's the Tokyo Marathon?" I found the training addictive. How much further could I go today? How much harder could I push myself? My only concern was my knees. They had never troubled me before but now I found some days after a long run I had trouble walking. My legs never ached; they were having the time of their lives on merry tours of Derbyshire. It felt like I was really achieving something, reclaiming my body from the disease.

I was also getting into the flow of things at work and felt like I knew more than when I went away. This was what I'd longed for. To be back as a member of the real world. But the happier I got, the more I feared the leukaemia coming back. I couldn't imagine going back to that dark place. But there was nothing I could do to insure against it, only live as though it would be back tomorrow.

February 2009

I'd been sweating profusely at night for a week before Mary told me to phone the hospital. We had both ignored the soaked sheets for that long. It simply wasn't convenient to believe anything could be wrong. Night sweats had been a feature of my illness before, so the return of any of the symptoms struck me cold.

I called the ward and told them the situation, asked them to put my mind at rest, knowing they could not. Come in for a blood test, they said. "When?" I said. "Now," they said. I looked at the clock. It was late morning, but what worried me was that it was a Friday. Significant things always happen to me on a Friday, and have throughout my life. The omens were bad. I put my hand to my head, unsure of what I was doing. "Look," I told Julie, the Assistant Editor, "I think I need to go. I've had a recurrence of a symptom I had when I was ill and they want me to come in for some tests." What could she say? She tried to reassure me and said take as long as I needed. She would see me later. I hoped beyond hope that that was true.

I drove to the hospital in a fog of anxiety, but I still believed I would be okay. I found my way to the haematology clinic and had my bloods taken, then went over to Mary's ward, where she was on shift. We didn't talk much. Her boss told her to go with me, they'd manage. We joked as we waited to see the doctor. I think we had to relieve the tension somehow. This was agonising. Eventually Dr. Woodward called us in. He was smiley and full of questions, which relaxed me a little. Maybe it was nothing after all. "It would be very unusual for it to be the leukaemia causing you to sweat," Dr. Woodward said. "I'd be very surprised if it was anything to worry about." He tapped my details into the computer. My results weren't on yet. He logged out and we talked for another couple of minutes and he examined me and listened to my chest. Then he checked the computer again. He tailed off the sentence and went quiet. The only sound his finger tapping beside the keys. I could spy one number on the screen lit in orange. The rest were green. It was my neutrophils. They were 0.7, meaning technically I was neutropenic i.e. in possession of a depleted immune system. I swallowed hard. "Oh," Dr. Woodward said, "well it could be your neutrophils are low because you're combating an infection. Have you felt unwell at all?" I shook my head. "I think what we should do is send you for a chest X-ray just to check there's nothing going on there infection-wise." I wasn't convinced but didn't believe it was the leukaemia. It just couldn't be. I was so well.

The X-ray waiting room was packed, and we had to wait for almost an hour before I was called. When I came back to the waiting room, Neville, the charge nurse from Mary's ward, was sitting with her. "They want you to stay in," Mary said, "because your counts are low, as a precaution while they find out what's wrong." My heart dropped into my shoes. This sounded serious. The thought of any more hospital time in my whole life made my head swim with disgust. I wondered how we'd got to this point so quickly, so without warning. My blood test just four weeks earlier had revealed nothing, suggested nothing but health. Now I was staring the worst in the face. But still I believed there would be an explanation.

We walked to a side room on Mary's ward and I perched on the bed. I felt like I was carrying a very heavy weight. I thought of my marathon, and the raw pain I would feel if it was taken away. Before long Dr. Cowdrey and Alison entered but still I thought nothing of it. I cracked a joke about them missing me and pulling strings to get me back. Neither laughed. "Richard," Dr. Cowdrey said, settling in the chair behind me, "we've had a look at the blood film and I'm afraid the blast cells are back again." "Oh my God," I heard Mary say as she seemed to deflate. The words hung there like an unexploded grenade, and I began to fold into myself, creasing and doubling towards the centre of pain. "I'm really very sorry,"Dr. Cowdrey said, putting his hand on my back. I began to cry uncontrollably, though, oddly, not for myself. I thought of my Mum, recently laid off from her job and so emotionally fragile anyway. I thought of my dad and Marion, my friends, how this would cut them in half. I felt like it was my fault, as though I'd dropped the ball somehow. Like a recovering alcoholic having to tell my family I was drinking again. I felt I'd let them down. They'd all got me back to health and I'd blown it.

"You're a young man," Dr. Cowdrey said. "There's no reason why we shouldn't try again. You will need a bone marrow transplant and probably two rounds of heavy chemotherapy before that." I closed my eyes, and all the memories of chemo came back in a surge. Could I go through that again? I didn't know. Dr. Cowdrey went on: "I've spoken to the doctors at Sheffield, which is where they do the transplants, and they suggested you have your treatment there. Sometimes the window for the transplant can be quite small so it makes sense if you are already there." I vaguely nodded my agreement. "It may be harder to get you into remission this time. The leukaemia is obviously more aggressive than we first thought and it may have returned with some mutations. I'm really very sorry," he said.

Dr. Cowdrey sent me home to grieve, and grieve is what I did. For the first couple of days I felt very fragile and struggled to summon any kind of strength or belief. "You've done it before, you can do it again," people said. I just sat there in the crater of the news, hopelessly lost and hopeless. I was going to have to get a handle on this somewhere, but I was simply stunned into nothingness. The worst had officially happened. My biggest fear was manifest. I knew that it was 50/50 this would happen, but I never, ever believed it would.

Over the few days that followed, though, I began to harden. Something was growing inside me. Faith? Resolve? I didn't know. But before I knew it, my game face was back. When bad news hits you, fear is an instant emotion, doubt an automatic response. But hope grows slower and, it grows stronger. I had learned not to chastise myself for feeling afraid. There's room for fear alongside belief. That's healthy. But never would I allow it to dominate me, to rule my emotions. If positivity counted for anything, and I believed it did, then I was going to have it on my side.

Course 5

Thursday February 12 2009. Course 5: Day 1: Chemo Day 1.

I returned to the Royal Hallamshire Hospital in Sheffield for my fifth course of chemotherapy. I was in determined mood and great shape physically. That had to count for something. But this was 'salvage' chemotherapy. It would be harsher and more demanding than anything I had been given before, including MACE, which had so horribly bleached my digestive system. The course of drugs I would have was known as Flag-Ida. The composite drugs were Fludarabine, which I hadn't had before, Cytarabine, which I'd had lots of, and Idarubicine, which was also new to me. Alongside these I would also receive GCSF injections, the bone marrow stimulant. It was a punishing regime over six days. After that, as before, my counts would drop and stay at zero for around two weeks before recovering. During my down time I would be an open door for infections. The worry was that the ward had two infections already doing the rounds, both of them nasty. One was the Norovirus, a vomiting and diarrhoea bug. The other, predictably, was C-diff. The superbug that stalked me but I had thus far side-stepped. I would be barrier-nursed to try and stop the passing of infection, but I knew these things tended to move freely from patient to patient. I was in a side room, which was a help. It was the Teen Suite, no less. I had internet access, in a fashion, which would be a nice novelty and would keep me more in touch with the world.

I was taken down to have a new Hickman line fitted, and couldn't believe how much smoother it went than the first time. The surgeon looked quizzically at my scar, then worked around it to insert the line pretty painlessly. That was a relief, and I hoped it would be a good omen for this treatment. I really should have known better by then.

I ran for the toilet and emptied out the contents of my stomach into the bowl, vomiting until there was nothing left to bring up. It was Day 1 of the drugs, and they had, it appeared, hit my stomach with full force. As was customary, I went right off food almost immediately, feeling unable to stomach anything. This was not the best start. To be so sick so early was definitely worrying because I had a long, long way to go. The doctors had told me that Flag-Ida often kept the counts down for longer. Plus, with the amount of chemotherapy I'd had, who could say how well I would recover from another bout. I had the impression I was in for a long haul.

Friday – Sunday: February 13 – 15 2009. Course 5: Days 2 - 4: Chemo Days 2 - 4.

Over the next couple of days the vomiting settled. I was still sick occasionally, but it was not as severe as I'd feared after Day 1. I ate what I felt able to keep down and my body began to find a rhythm with the toxic liquids being pumped around my veins. One of the Flag-Ida drugs was known to be toxic to the heart, so I had been sent for a cardiac echo to check my heart was going to be able to take the strain. They must have decided it was, because we pressed ahead.

I got the feeling this was kitchen sink therapy the best weapon they had for where I was. But I don't think I really took stock of how serious the situation had become. I had relapsed and relapsed quickly. The leukaemia was now likely to be resistant, to some degree, to chemotherapy. A remission now would be hard won. But I was ploughing on, day to day, somehow in the belief that not much had changed or the same rules applied.

People would ask me how I got through the days with the awful gravity of death on my back. There are three answers to that. The first is belief – trusting I would beat the odds. The second is a kind of denial simply refusing to think on things too deeply, acting as though all of this was some abysmal package holiday. The third is that, sometimes, I didn't cope. I got upset or, more commonly, became very introverted and distant. Mary kept me afloat when I started to let in water, but, I should say, this was happening less at that stage than it did during earlier treatment. My spirits were fairly high most of the time, and I felt a renewed appetite for the fight, if not for food. I had been puzzling over the question whether my past bout with the disease had made me a stronger person, or whether it had taken something from me. I might have given different answers on different days. The verdict I settled on was that, in my case, I felt it had made me stronger. But its effects were more far-reaching. I felt new levels of empathy and my enjoyment of things had sharpened somehow. I was less patient, less content to be idle. And I seemed to have developed a much more assertive personality. If someone could facilitate something for me I'd just come out and ask for it. If I wasn't satisfied with something, I'd say so. I was never rude; I was just taking ownership of my life. But there was little living going on where I was then. The days would grind by painfully slowly.

Mary and I would mop up all the laughs that were to be had but there weren't many. I struggled with sickness and a lingering, background curtain of nausea which, despite my best efforts, stole a lot of the wind from my sails. Even as the run of drugs came to an end, the feeling of sickness persisted. But, aside from the odd bout of vomiting, it was manageable. I found mints to be a help, in keeping the sickness at bay, but other suggested remedies like ginger biscuits, didn't work for me. Distractions were important too. I had developed a minor obsession with *Connect4*, and none of my visitors escaped without a game. I taught Mary to play chess, which she didn't much enjoy, but it was an hour killed and many more of them had to be despatched before sundown. We also dabbled with draughts, something Mary turned out to play a bit too well. She was like *Rainman*. We didn't play again.

February 2009

My counts were coming down steadily but so, unfortunately, was my weight. Each morning my bloods would be taken and I would be invited to sit in the weighing chair. The results of each chartered a steady decline. The first thing the body converts into energy, because it finds it easier to do so, is muscle mass. It broke my heart to watch all that strength I had slogged and sweated for melt away in a matter of weeks. I had built myself up from nothing over the course of my recovery. Now I was sliding back towards the brink and I couldn't watch. I rarely looked in a mirror. I sunk below 11 stone in a matter of days and the weight continued to fall away, like sand in an egg timer. I knew an infection was probably in the post. My neutrophils were zero and I'd never dodged one yet. I just had to hope it would be a minor bug.

The first to arrive was fairly pedestrian, but then I compared everything to the ESBL that nearly killed me. I was on antibiotics for about a week, and felt pretty unwell for a few days, but the infection packed up and left with little argument. I'd have been very contented had that been as bad as it got, but it wasn't to be. Before too long, my blood cultures showed up another E-coli bug. The doctors told me it was a pretty nasty one and I would need to have some similarly nasty antibiotics. After trying a couple of different treatments, they eventually settled on Septrin, a particularly unpleasant but effective antibiotic. Septrin has the added side effect of inducing nausea, something I didn't need as my weight sunk below 10 stone. It was also known to impede the recovery of blood counts, meaning I faced spending even longer in hospital. But I had no choice in the matter, and things were about to get worse in any case.

My stool sample tested positive for both C-diff and the Norovirus, the two outbreaks on the ward. When the doctors told me this little titbit of news, I laughed. It was an involuntary action. I just found it funny somehow that my luck could be so conspicuously absent. I could be treated for C-diff with oral antibiotics, but there was no treatment for the Norovirus, which just had to be ridden out. My main worry now was how much weight I was going to lose.

I still had nausea from my chemo drugs, added to by the antibiotics. Then there was the Norovirus, which was characterised by projectile vomiting. There seemed little chance of me holding on to much weight at all, which was bad news heading, as I was, into transplant. Mary and I looked at each other and did the only thing we could. We played *Connect4*.

At first the changes were subtle, I noticed that typing out text messages on my phone had become harder. I kept catching the wrong keys or pressing them too many times. I didn't really pay much attention. I was feeling pretty unwell and suffering from my usual mild hallucinations, which made my hands or the room feel huge or tiny. It was nothing in the grand scheme of things, although my Mum was becoming concerned about the stray consonants littering my replies, as though I was sending her *Countdown conundrums*.

The problem didn't come to a head until a day or two later when I lost the ability to read. I was going through the day's newspaper when, suddenly, the letters melted and jumbled and merged. I blinked hard at the page to see the letters all looked alien, a mass of squiggles and blotches. I knew then something was seriously wrong. I pressed my buzzer and told the nurse what was happening, though my words were beginning to fail me and I couldn't swallow. She left me to go and buzz the doctor. I picked up the phone and called Mary. It was 11 p.m. She got in the car and set off. I was going downhill fast. I could manage to speak only by concentrating very hard, but one side of my face had fallen. The doctor on call arrived and began asking me questions and making me push against him with both arms and legs. I could do what he asked of me, but I was terrified I was having a stroke, all the symptoms were there.

By the time Mary got to me I'd lost control of my hands. They'd curled up tightly and were fixed under my chin. The doctors were convinced that I wasn't having a stroke. It was a reaction to the drugs and I had become very agitated, which was preventing me getting a grip on my faculties. Mary tried to calm me down, and I found I could overcome some of the problems if I really concentrated. I was prescribed Zopiclone, a powerful sedative, and had one right away. Over the next hour, things began to return to normal and I was soothed back down from the sky. Mary told me later, as I drifted off to sleep, I was laughing uncontrollably about something.

Being sent for an MRI scan was a welcome escape from the ward. Doctors were checking that last night's episode hadn't caused any damage to my brain. I relished getting off the ward. I was neutropenic and being barrier-nursed for C-diff and Norovirus, I wasn't allowed out of my room ordinarily. I couldn't even stretch my legs in the hallway. Consequently I was going stir-crazy in my room. Being fenced in by those four walls and the steady repetition of the days were gnawing away at my sanity. I had served more than three weeks in isolation, not leaving the ward once, other than for a fire drill which, again, perversely, I quite enjoyed.

I would gaze out of my tower block window at the streets below, at the tiny figures going about their lives as though the ability to do so was a given. Some days I still couldn't believe I was up to my neck in all of this. But then, I was always getting myself into mad situations, finding myself trapped inside anecdotes. I got run over by a bus once. A naked gypsy child once urinated all over my shoes. Stuff like that just kind of happened to me. Granted, this was a little more grave, but I had some stories to tell all the same. Now I just had to live to tell them. Another day, another expensive medical procedure. The MRI was clear. My brain was undamaged. We were relieved, of course. You had to give thanks for each mercy. I had my attention fixed on getting home from that point on. I was nowhere near well enough at that moment and my counts were returning very slowly. But I was getting myself in the right frame of mind, warning my body that I still had certain expectations of it, despite everything. Mary told me not to put too much pressure on myself or rush things. I had to be sure I had shaken off all my infections. I knew all that but being in that room was beginning to feel like an itch I couldn't scratch.

March 2009

Three weeks became four. It was now officially the longest stint I had done in hospital. It was hardly surprising; the whole course had felt like we were pushing against something, sailing into a head wind. But I was a seasoned pro now though, right? This was all I knew for six months. It was true that I was possessed with more knowledge about my disease, my treatment, and all the drugs on offer. That definitely was a plus. I could give doctors a précis on exactly how I felt, when asked, knowing what was important and what I would just have to live with. It was altogether an easier place to be than that first course forever ago, during which I understood little of what was happening to me. I also knew I was closing in on getting out of there, so I stepped up my strategy. My plan was two-fold, both strands of which boiled down to lying. Essentially, when I saw a doctor I would perk myself right up, and affect the manner of a person much healthier than I genuinely felt. I smiled. I told them I felt good, thank you for asking. When asked if I'd vomited or had diarrhoea, I answered no. Now this is a rather serious porky pie if you get it wrong. I did not have diarrhoea, that was true. It was occasional. So was the vomiting, but I felt, in myself, that things were picking up sufficiently that I could leave. I just had to get their feelings in line with my own. It took a couple of days to achieve that, but I got Dr. Dobson, one of the consultants, to agree I could go home if my counts made similar improvements to the day previously. I needed a neutrophil count of 1.0 to be allowed out. When they came in at 1.7, I shouted "Yes" loud enough to be heard right down the ward.

I waited patiently to be told I could leave, for a few hours I waited before losing composure. I stopped a junior doctor outside my room. Her reply completely sunk me. They wanted me to stay another night to check it wasn't a fluke result. I was having the GCSF injections, which could have inflated the result significantly. I skulked back to my room, crestfallen. The need to get out of their swells to such an extent that it's all you can think about. I sat in my room for a few minutes before deciding I didn't agree with the decision. I went and found the doctor again and laid on what is surely the biggest guilt-trip any human has ever been subjected to. I told her how desperate I was to get out, how my counts were far in excess of the 1.0 reading required and how Dr. Dobson had promised I could leave with such improvements. She tried to take it all in, before saying she would pass on my concerns to Dr. Dobson after he had finished the meeting he was currently in. I returned to my room, satisfied that I'd given it everything I had.

About an hour later I was cleared to leave. We bundled my stuff together with infinitely more excitement than we had packed it and waited for my medications to be sent from pharmacy. While we waited, I was sick, quite violently. Mary freaked out a little. Should I really be doing this? It was the tail- end of the Norovirus, I said. That was probably the last of it. I wasn't strong enough to walk out, I left, bashed but unbroken, in a wheelchair pushed by my good wife.

Previously, on my release, I was possessed by a ravenous hunger as my body fought to reload the weight I had lost. For the first few days, this was lacking. I ate, sure enough, but I was picking at things and leaving half portions. I felt sick and had to keep dosing myself up on anti-emetics. Occasionally, I would crumble into projectile vomiting and I felt extremely tired, often sleeping through half the afternoon. It was hell for Mary, who wrestled with the compulsion to phone the hospital. But I would always talk her down. Tomorrow things will settle. Despite the scares, things were improving slightly and I knew we had an appointment at Chesterfield in a few days for a bone marrow biopsy, where we could ask for any advice on my condition.

When that day came I was starting to pick up. I was able to walk a lot more strongly and didn't feel so sick. We asked Alison about my vomiting and she didn't seem too concerned. "We'll get you some more anti-sickness drugs together before you leave," she said. Pained slightly, all I had to get through now was the bone marrow biopsy, a procedure I didn't relish. I lay down on my front trying to remember how many of them I'd had. I wasn't sure. Dr. Woodward carried it out very quickly and smoothly. "We've got a good sample there," he said, showing me the specks of my marrow spread out on a dish. "That's usually a good sign." I prayed he was right as I lay there alone in the treatment room, putting pressure on the red, felt-tip dot of a wound.

Just as my hunger began to return I encountered another problem. Diarrhoea. At first it was occasional, before long I was going several times in the night. We both agreed I should phone the hospital to ask advice, though I was frozen by the fear of going back. Luckily the doctor just advised me to keep an eye on it, drink lots of fluids, phone back if it got worse. Unfortunately, the next day, it got worse.

Tuesday March 24 2009. Course 5: Day 41.

I called again and was told to come in for a check-over and to give a sample. There was a bed for me on E-floor, as Ward P3 was full. We sombrely packed a bag and drove in to Sheffield. I lifted the bag into hospital, evidence I was getting stronger, and studied the board. E-floor – Infectious Diseases and Tropical Medicines. I chuckled to myself. Where to put the lad with low immunity? I might turn up with diarrhoea and leave with yellow fever.

E-floor was not the swishly refurbished unit up on P-floor. It was dark and old fashioned and everything had a sign on it warning not to touch it. The staff had that glazed-over look only the unsatisfied can master. I was shown to a side room that was equally depressing and oddly quiet. There we waited for a doctor to take my bloods and I gave them a sample, the results of which wouldn't be available for a couple of days so I hoped my release wouldn't depend on them. My blood results showed a worrying drop in neutrophils from 1.7 when I left hospital to 0.6. Fighting off a bug could account for some of that but not all. I didn't give much thought to what it might mean. I made the mistake of asking the same junior doctor if she knew the results of my bone marrow. She froze and I saw it. "I know the consultants have made a finding but I can't really ... you'd have questions and I'm not the right person to answer them. Sorry, I just can't tell you." I swallowed. My gut instinct, from her reaction, was 'no remission'. Mary's was too, although she tried to put a gloss on it. We were sent home again, as my blood test showed no infection, but I was laden with a doubt about what I would be told on Monday. I tried not to think on it too much but, for the remaining days, my smile had a puncture.

I hadn't had many dealings with Carl Dobson, the other consultant haematologist at the Hallamshire. I was surprised when I first heard he was a consultant, only because he seemed very young. But what did I know? You only got to that position on merit. It was Dr. Dobson who stood at the foot of my bed that Monday afternoon. He was joined by Dr. Peters, and Hayley Jackson one of the transplant co-ordinators. Alarm bells began to ring in my head. It was never good news when the whole gang came in to deliver it. I expected to be told that I wasn't in remission but it was much worse than that.

In the conversation that followed, Dr. Dobson used the word 'difficult' at least ten times. We were in a 'difficult' situation, I had a 'difficult' leukaemia, a 'difficult' decision had to be made. The treatment I had just received, Flag-Ida, itself a heavy duty regime, had had little effect Dr. Dobson told me. My leukaemia had shrunk fairly significantly from around a 90% concentration in my bone marrow to around 30%. But this was a far greater number of cells to have survived for the chemotherapy to have been called a success. A treatment as robust as I'd just undergone should have induced a remission, less than 5% of cancerous cells remaining, or at least a near remission. I was hit by a wave of despair as it became truly clear, perhaps for the first time, that I might not beat this thing. "We are at the stage," Dr. Dobson said, "where it would be wrong for us to press ahead with more treatment, without offering you the choice to … " he paused, "to go down the other road and not undergo further chemotherapy, knowing that it might not be effective." I felt my head swell with emotion. I was too ill, too weak, too tired to handle news like that. I composed myself enough to ask, "What chance do I have of beating this now?" Dr. Dobson sighed, "I would say, on balance, your chances of still being here in five years are about 15%." That statement was particularly barbed. He went on, "If you chose to continue treatment we would support you 100%. The regime would involve very high doses of Cytarabine, in a bid to get you back into remission, or, more likely, clear the bone marrow altogether. The chances of getting that result, are, maybe 50-50. Then you would, of course, need to receive radiotherapy and a transplant. You need to understand that that course of action would be likely to make you very ill and it carries a substantial morbidity rate." I caught sight of Mary, sitting opposite me, very alone in a plastic chair, her face striped with tears. She didn't deserve this. I didn't care about myself any more; not my ravaged body or scarred mind, but I couldn't do something so callous as to die.

"I think perhaps you need time to think about what I've just told you, Dr. Dobson said. "You could go home tonight and have a talk, but if you wanted to continue treatment then obviously we would want to start quickly. You could have another Hickman line fitted tomorrow, as we had originally planned." The team shuffled out as Mary and I gathered our belongings in a detached way, as though clearing a house after a death. We somehow made it through the corridors and down to the car, where Mary phoned her mum to tell her the news. She replied, simply, "Come home."

It just didn't seem real. I couldn't come to terms with what had been said. I had done the treatment, and everything that had been asked of me, but now it seemed the leukaemia had stepped up its bid to take me. It had stopped playing by the rules. Mary and I talked it over and both felt the same, stopping treatment could not be dismissed, it had to be discussed. But, as we talked about it, that seemed inherently wrong to us both. After all we had faced, after all we had lost, to give in now and, in a sense, to give up on each other, was something we couldn't do.

Everyone else we consulted said the same; "It is your decision and we will support you either way." But their eyes said "fight", and our hearts did too. It was a hard decision but an easy one all the same. If that's how the disease wanted to play it, then I would respond in kind giving myself the highest dose chemotherapy I could realistically survive. My old thoughts about the marathon came back to me, "Even if it gets me in the end, I want it to know it's been in a fight." My initial fear turned to determination, then a boiling anger. I was a young man, a good person, I was in love. How dare it try to take that from me? This would be, I knew, the hardest thing I would ever have to go through. I knew the treatment would take me to the edge of death, and I would, at times, wish I was dead. But the sicker I got, the sicker the leukaemia would become. We were going on a little trip together, and only one of us would be coming back. In a strange sort of way, I was looking forward to it.

Wednesday March 25 2009. Course 5: Day 42.

The following morning, I arrived at the Hallamshire early, joining once again the dark queue to have a Hickman line fitted. My last one had been removed swiftly as a possible cause of infection, although I don't think it was ever confirmed as being responsible. One thing that I can say about the Hallamshire, they were always quick to whip out a Hickman line at the merest suggestion there could be a problem with it. They were a little trigger-happy with them at times.

I was given two units of blood, my red cell count having dropped to 7.5. A nurse told me that my consultants, Drs. Snell and Dobson, had been reading research papers and making enquiries, trying to ensure they put me on the regime which seemed to have the best chance of success. It boiled down to a choice between super-high doses of Cytarabine alone, or super-high doses of Cytarabine, coupled with Mitoxantrone. In the end, the doctors decided my best chance was to have both; the Mitoxantrone alongside the Cytarabine sledge-hammer. I was happy with that decision. I would have drunk rat-poison if they told me it might help. I had nine days of chemo ahead. The strongest stuff they had. The atom bomb of chemotherapy, and fallout was to be expected. Dr. Snell had warned me that 20 percent of patients receiving what I was about to receive would die of the toxicity of the treatment or complications thereof. The side effects would be the same as before, probably worse. I was told there would be a 'significant' risk of brain or other organ damage. I listened carefully to all the pitfalls of pressing ahead, but nothing could have changed my mind. I signed the form. "Do your worst," I told Dr. Peters. She gave me a half smile, and I knew right then it would be worse than I could imagine.

Course 6

Friday March 26 2009. Course 6: Day 1: Chemo Day 1.

I was more than a little hacked-off that I was only given tablet anti-sickness drugs to begin with. If you are on high dose chemotherapy, IV anti-emetics are a must. I consider myself to have a fairly strong stomach, but it was no match for this new drug regime which I later learned was four times the dose of anything I'd had before.

Once you start with vomiting, it's a tricky cycle to break. I began right away. If you can't keep anything down you physically will not have the strength to come through it. My weight was down to begin with, so I was going to need help. The idea of a nasal-gastric (or NG) tube had been discussed to help supplement my nutrition. This involved having a tube inserted through the nose and down the throat into the stomach. The end would sit there, taped to my face, and provide a port through which they could feed me a kind of mushed-up soup of a mixture. A junior doctor appeared in the doorway carrying the apparatus. I sighed. At least it was another procedure I could tick off in my *Top Trumps* arsenal. The initial thrust up the nostril is fairly unpleasant, but I managed to tolerate the rest of it with minimal gagging. The tube itself wasn't as slim as I'd hoped it might me, so it felt like exactly what it was a tube stuck in your throat. "You'll get more used to it," they said. As it turned out, I only had to put up with it for a couple of hours. Spun by nausea, I was sick again, so violently, I'd vomited out the entire tube, which I am assured is quite hard to do. It was removed. "We'll try again another time," they said, "once we get on top of the vomiting."

Monday March 30 2009. Course 6: Day 4: Chemo Day 4.

By now, I felt like a ghost. I'd hardly eaten a thing and the weight was falling off me at an unprecedented rate. I just wanted to curl into a ball and do nothing. It felt like I was being eaten away from the inside each time my veins were flooded with poison.

I had an appointment to see Dr. Dobbs at Weston Park Hospital, to make the arrangements for my radiotherapy sessions. Weston Park was just around the corner, but I was to be taken there in a medical taxi a ride which would surely last no longer than a minute. I didn't protest. I was half-hoping for a piggy-back down the corridor. The receptionist didn't seem sure where to send us and we ended up traipsing round several departments, which left me feeling increasingly drained.

By the time we reached the right ward I was really nagging. Mary implored one of the nurses to help me and he showed us to a side room in which we could wait in private. He gave me a cardboard tray in case I felt sick. I filled it, incidentally, just as Dr. Dobbs walked in. "Oh dear," she said, by way of a greeting, and I sensed I was not the first patient she had walked in on mid-puke. She skipped asking me how I was feeling, and we got down to the matter in hand. Radiotherapy was needed to destroy my bone marrow and immune system. The transplant would then have a blank canvas on which to engraft. The transplanted stem cells find their way from the bloodstream into the bone marrow. Boffins still don't know how they do this. Once there, they begin to generate a new immune system, the donor's to be exact. This is where complications can and do arise. The new and what's left of the old immune systems recognise each other as foreign and square up. The result is Graft Versus Host Disease (GVHD), which is a funny old thing. Those with it could exhibit a wide range of symptoms, and these could persist for a long time or only surface several years down the line. The benefit of this new immune system is that it targets what is left of the cancerous cells, rather than accommodating them like the old system did. It is only capable of destroying a small number of cancerous cells, however, which is why a transplant patient really needs to be in remission when the process starts. If the cancer has too strong a foothold it will overwhelm the new immune system and you will die anyway. You need a bit of GVHD to fight the leukaemia, but too much will attack your organs and kill you. Drugs are given to try and regulate the extent of GVHD you have but it's not an exact science.

The radiotherapy treatment itself would take place inside a large room which looked like a cross between a recording studio and a nuclear reactor. I was to lie sideways-on to the machine, and be bombarded with rays. My head and organs would be protected by brass plates hanging between me and the machine. I would go through the process every day for four days, during which I would stay at Weston Park. The range of side effects attached to radiotherapy were dizzying. They seemed to incorporate all those which were part and parcel of chemo, and then many more besides. The most daunting of these seemed to be the stripping of the soft tissue of the digestive tract, meaning painful blisters from mouth through to bottom. This was said to be so uncomfortable many patients were on constant morphine infusions. It was clear why some patients, particularly older ones, refused treatment when told they need chemotherapy and radiotherapy. In my mind the path of treatment was preferable to death. But only just. I looked again at Dr. Dobbs, a tall and slight woman who looked more librarian than anything else. But she was an intelligent and compassionate woman. That much was obvious. I felt I could trust her. If I could get a remission from this round of chemo, I had a chance of beating it for good. Even if the path led through the valley in the shadow of death.

April 2009

As I was in hospital and incapable of doing so myself, Mary took on board the financial running of the Woolley Household Plc. As if she didn't have enough to do as my full time carer, secretary, cheer leader and saviour. As was inevitable, we were beginning to have more going out than we were coming in. My wages had dropped to three-quarters of my usual pay and were due to drop to half-pay the following month. My employers had been fantastic in that respect paying me for far longer than I was contracted for. But I had exhausted the system, as had Mary, whose wage had been zero for some time.

Worse was to come though as Mary's boss called her in for a meeting with HR about 'the future'. We had bigger things to worry about, but Mary was upset, sensing they were going to try and force her out. She was right, as it turned out. They asked her to give a date on which she intended to return to work. With the circumstances as they were, this was something she couldn't do. Nothing was certain in our lives at that moment. "Well," they said, "you leave us with no choice but to terminate your contract. Either that or you could agree to take a career break." Don't it make your heart glow with the milk of human kindness.

We were unsure what a career break meant exactly, but it sounded instantly better than the sack. It entailed, we learned, leaving her post indefinitely, leaving the payroll, therefore freeing up a position which could be filled with someone not going through some kind of crisis. But, it meant leaving on the proviso that a job, of some kind, would be found for her at such a time as she felt able to return. This guarantee seemed paper-thin, based on the word of people we had lost respect for. "It was a simple numbers situation, "they said. They needed to fill the holes in the rota with people who were going to be there. Nothing personal. Just personnel.

Mary was sent away from the office, sobbing, to 'consider her options'. Everyone she told was furious. It just didn't seem fair or right. Was it even legal, we wondered? We read through Mary's contract and asked the advice of a solicitor friend and came to the conclusion that it was, sadly, within their power. The NHS is a wonderful, wonderful thing I will defend to my grave. But while they're prolific in looking after the vulnerable, they don't seem so good at looking after themselves.

We were used to being asked to make decisions that seemed to lead to dire resolutions on both sides. But, once again, there was an obviously preferably option. To appeal against a sacking would mean several meetings with boards who would almost certainly uphold the decision anyway. Her future career at the hospital would probably suffer if she kicked up a fuss, as tempting as it was. I suppose that's how they get you. Catch 22. Mary agreed she would begin a career break in a few weeks' time, after being remunerated for holidays she hadn't taken. I think it hurt Mary more than she let on. All around us people were contorting themselves to help us however they could, but here there was someone pulling the rug from under us.

The only other obstinate party was our mortgage lender, our biggest outgoing of course. We had contacted them on the advice of more than one financial advisor and been assured they were duty-bound to help us. Their governing body simply does not allow them to shut the door on borrowers caught out in the cold of a miserable recession. Now, whether to name and shame this mortgage lender. Since they did me no favours, I'm reluctant to do them one. I had asked the Nationwide, for it was she, if we could switch to interest-only payments. We didn't have enough equity in the property and hadn't been paying for long enough to be considered for that. I explained the difficulty of our circumstances again. Could an exception be made? No, they said. They offered me the chance to extend the term of the mortgage, until Mary was 75 or something similar, but even this only reduced the monthly payments by something negligible. "The only other thing we can suggest is for you to sign a declaration that you cannot keep up with the repayments and we will negotiate a more attainable figure with you." I laughed. "And that would destroy our credit references, wouldn't it?" "They would be affected, yes," they said. The conversation had hit a dead end. Mary probably would have gone ahead with their suggestion if I'd wanted to, but I didn't want to torpedo both our hopes of ever getting credit again. Anyway, we'd get by, somehow. It's not like I was expecting anything more. Ever hear of anyone with a good word to say about a bank?

My condition had been worsening on all fronts for some time before they made the call. I suppose they don't send you to Intensive Care on a whim. My temperature had blasted through 40°C and I sunk under a very heavy fever, flavoured with various hallucinations. I remember writhing around on the bed and must have been speaking in tongues because a doctor tried to calm me down. "Richard, do you know where you are?" he asked. "Yes," I said eventually, "but I think I should be in hospital instead." If this surprised or tickled him, he didn't react. "Where do you think you are?" I shifted on the bed. "I'm on the set of Emmerdale, wherever they film that. Leeds sort of way." The doctor perched on the edge of my bed. A young man, kindly, black-rimmed spectacles. "Richard," he said, "you <u>are</u> in hospital. You're on ITU because you're very poorly. But you're here so we can keep a closer eye on you. You're going to be okay." When I next nodded into consciousness, he was gone. The funny thing is, I can't be sure whether he existed at all.

Mary's birthday came and went with me in ITU. I didn't manage to pick her up a present, probably the only time I would ever get away with it. I really was sinking at that point and was once again tormented by dreams I thought to be real. I dreamed I was to be tried for two famous murders. I can only recall one of them specifically, that of OJ Simpson's wife. I felt guilty of, or at least complicit in, these murders and was terrified of being convicted. I remember having a long conversation with my dad during which he had to reassure me I didn't have any upcoming court appearances. But worse still were the dreams that Mary had left me, that she had another man now and had very coldly severed all ties with me. I had lost my grip on time so couldn't say for how long I believed this to be true, but it was the most agonising period of my life.

The doctors were having trouble pinning down exactly what was wrong with me, but it was looking certain that I had some kind of lung infection. Just as a precaution, they whipped my Hickman line out again. But my temperatures were persisting and my breathing was getting worse, meaning I now needed oxygen by mask. The doctors rubbed their chins and decided what I really needed at that stage of my life was one of the most unpleasant waking procedures out there. A bronchoscopy. A team made up of a surprisingly high number of medical staff surround your bed and shove a succession of swabs and cameras down your throat. "Try not to gag," they told me beforehand. I gagged my way through the whole thing, but they told me I'd tolerated it quite well at the end. I'd obviously pissed someone off somewhere because I also had a bone marrow biopsy that day. That would tell us if this atom bomb chemo had worked. If my bone marrow wasn't empty, it was all over.

I was pretty much out-of-it when they put in my chest drain, so I can't really tell you what it's like. It's basically a catheter that drains fluid out of the chest. Mine didn't last long, it fell out. I had never really rejoined the land of the living and my blood pressure and temperature were still all over the place. So, at precisely midnight of my birthday, I was sent back to ITU. Mary was told at this point that I had pneumonia, but I don't remember being privy to that information. However, they could have told me they'd discovered my DNA was identical to an elephant's and I was to be known as Nellie until the end of my days, and I would have just pulled the same face and remembered as much of it.

Though I didn't know it at the time, I was in a lot of trouble. I had no immune system, was painfully weak and I had pneumonia. All this brought us to a difficult crossroads. My bone marrow result had indeed come back empty, the outcome we were praying for. But it was all for nothing if I was to die in the coming days, which was looking increasingly likely. The doctors had one last trump card up their sleeve, my own stem cells, harvested back in December. They had the potential to regenerate my own immunity and, alongside a trolley-full of antibiotics and drugs, might be enough to get me out the other side. So, on my birthday, I was given the gift of my stem cells back.

Harvesting them had been an entirely optional procedure, which some of my doctors had called a waste of time. But here I was needing them very badly indeed. It was a strange thing, having them back, being my own donor. All my family who visited during the transfusion were greeted with the strongest smell of sweetcorn. That's what they smell like, the transplant nurses said. Although, you can't smell your own. This was true, I couldn't smell a thing.

I spent another day on ITU, before being moved back to P3. Writing this, I am aware that putting down every medical detail of my experiences would be boring, first and foremost, and secondly a little unsavoury. But I think it important I speak the truth and do not just glaze over some of the dirty details. I may as well tell you, therefore, that I was totally incontinent by this stage. I had a catheter fitted which carried away my fluids, but from the other end, I had very little control or notice over when something may be coming. I once soiled myself while my dad was sitting by my bedside. I didn't see any benefit in telling him, though I knew he would understand. Sometimes I would have presence to ask for a bedpan, but this was scarcely less humiliating than not bothering. The nursing staff were always exemplary in their treatment of me, but a lot of my cleaning and bed changing was done by Mary. We both preferred it that way. I'm telling you this because it may help to explain some of my behaviour later on, to explain more what the days were like and where I was sliding to mentally.

On ITU I had been visited by a psychiatrist who had talked to me about my feelings and coping mechanisms. He offered me anti-depressants, something I instinctively declined. I was not the sort of person who took anti-depressants whatever the circumstances. I was quite indignant at the time and didn't even consider it.

Later, Mary and others suggested giving them a go. I think they recognised I was sinking lower than I had before and maybe needed a little help. They were right, I reasoned, and asked for the prescription to be drawn up.

Friday – Sunday: April 24 - 26 2009. Course 6: Days 29 - 31.

Over the next few days there were going to be a tough couple of events to negotiate emotionally. The first was the bone marrow donor session, organised primarily by Mary's Auntie Sheila and a neighbour of hers, but contributed to by a lot of others. I had written a press release about it and my friends in the local papers did a great job in promoting it for us. Flyers had gone up round the village of Tibshelf and a Facebook group had been created for the cause but we still didn't know how many would attend. I had wanted to go but, obviously, my health made that impossible. In a way though, I felt it might be better I not go. I did not want to be a poster-boy for the day and the event was not about me. We were not looking for donors for me, but for others. I was most clear about that. Thanks to the Anthony Nolan Trust staff and all the helpers on the day, the event was a great success. A total of 53 new names were added to the register, some of them my old school friends or team-mates from football. God bless you all.

The second emotional hurdle came just days later, on Sunday, April 26. The London Marathon. A day I had run over in my mind a thousand times, a day I had poured my heart into. It was meant to be a day of hope and inspiration, which of course it was for so many, just not for me. I felt physically crushed by the irony of it all. I believed I should be there bouncing on the start line, hungry to get away and prove something to myself, to cancer and to everyone who doubted me. Instead I lay crippled in a hospital bed watching the damn thing on TV. Of all the things leukaemia had taken from me, this was among the most painful. Watching the start of the race left me with an awful crawling in my stomach, like a foot-long worm that writhed and gnawed on my insides. It was only because I had four family members running that I bothered to watch at all. "Next year, you'll be there," people told me. I nodded vaguely in agreement, but it was hard to escape the feeling that this was an opportunity missed, my opportunity taken away. I was filled with an icy feeling that I would never get a chance to run again.

April 2009

Each day was a horribly drawn-out affair. It was now day 33 of this chemo regime, the longest straight run I had spent in hospital by more than a week. I was hardly eating, sleeping in snatches and had the worst diarrhoea you could imagine. The chemo had been, as promised, truly awful. It had stripped and bleached everything out of me and I was left a shadow, or rather, a skeleton, of my former self. There was some good news, my neutrophils had reached 0.1. Nothing to crow about ordinarily, but in my case, it was my stem cells kicking in, the cavalry. Still, I felt rotten, physically and mentally. I kept crying and asking people to help me, and they would return kindly stares, though there was nothing anyone could do.

The horrible crawly feeling of chemo and recovery is something you simply can't describe to anyone else. I felt completely alien in my own body. I could never settle, was never the right temperature, was never comfortable. It's like you're desperately trying to shed your skin like a snake, but you can't get out of it. That feeling, minute by minute, day on day, makes you want to die. It feels like the only release. I kept crying and still asking people to help me, and they continued to return kindly stares, though there was nothing anyone could do.

May 2009

The chest drain was returned to the left of my back. If I recall correctly it drained about a litre of fluid very fast. For about a week, they opened the tap daily and something like 3.5 litres came out of my chest. Better out than in, when it came to my pneumonia it seemed.

My neutrophils had climbed to 0.4, quite a useful number when you're used to nothing. Still, it was another agonising nine days in the furnace before the doctors decided to carry out another bone marrow biopsy, to check the leukaemia was still absent. The results came back more or less empty of cells, which was good news. Could they think about sending me home then? I was so desperate to get out of there, though I was scared about how I would cope on the outside world. My weight was around 8 stone 6 lbs. and I could hardly stand or walk. I was still on oxygen round the clock. It seemed as though I would never be well enough to leave. I couldn't imagine ever feeling normal again.

Friday May 22 2009. Course 6: Day 57.

But, mercifully, the day came when they agreed I could go. There were conditions attached. I would be staying at Mary's mum's house, where there was a bed and a shower on the ground floor. I was to continue on the oxygen for as long as needed and would need visits from nurses and physios on a regular basis. Had Mary not been a nurse I don't think they would have let me go when they did. Had I not clearly been so desperate to get out I think they would have kept me longer still. But, after 57 straight days in hospital, I was sent home in a rickety old ambulance. To begin with I felt every bump of Sheffield's streets under the wheels, but soon I was asleep, to the amazement of the ambulance crew. Perhaps it was the relief of escape that soothed me into slumber despite the bumpy ride.

What Happened Next

Richard's journal stops here with his last entry on Friday 22 May 2009 after he is discharged from hospital following his sixth course of chemotherapy at the Royal Hallamshire Hospital.

What follows is a summary of what happened after that, plus some comments to fill gaps left in the journal itself so that the reader can get a fuller picture.

May & June 2009

Richard's weight was frighteningly low when he was allowed home from hospital. His mind and determination had suffered enormously and his discharge came at a time when we all doubted whether he would be able to come back from the abyss once again. Ann and John's home was kitted out like a hospital room, there was so much equipment and goodness knows how many different types of drugs present. With love and support around the clock from Mary and her mum, Richard slowly returned to us. He encountered further problems along the way, such as almost losing sight in an eye due to the various infections he still experienced.

A further bone marrow biopsy revealed that Richard was still in remission, and all stops were pulled out to find a matching bone marrow donor so that Richard could receive a life-saving transplant. The main transplant donor registers used by hospitals are: The Anthony Nolan Trust, The NHS Blood Service, a small register in Wales, European Register (predominantly made up of Germans or so we believe), and one in the United States.

The British based ones are searched first. Incredibly, almost all of the population of Germany is automatically signed up for the donor register, as they have to opt out, rather than in this country where we have to opt in. Therefore our numbers are depressingly low. Thankfully, we understood that a female donor was found on the Anthony Nolan register.

There is much that any donor has to sacrifice in respect of time to prepare for what is expected of them, drugs to receive, and the stem cells to harvest, when they volunteer to be a donor. Their reward is knowing that they may give someone they will never meet the gift of life. Is it possible to give anything more than that? The donor was put on standby on several occasions, but Richard's health was not yet ready for the transplant. Richard and Mary were still having meetings with the transplant team at the Hallamshire in June 2009.

Soon after, Richard and Mary were told the leukaemic cells were back. This meant that the aggressive nature of the leukaemia had won out against all the NHS could throw at it. Long meetings were held with Dr. Snell and his team. The outcome was that there was nothing more that could be done to remove the leukaemia; the transplant, so long the potential saviour, was cancelled as this would now be pointless; and the only realistic thing left to do was to go home and try and enjoy life as much as possible for what remained. The obvious question was asked by Richard himself – How long? – The answer was months only, certainly not years.

When news that his leukaemia was diagnosed as terminal, it was clear he would not be returning to work. His employer had been magnificent throughout his illness, but they still decided to beat anything they had done before. He was immediately put back on to full-pay, the gratitude to them we all feel is immeasurable. We were in regular contact with his Editor, Amanda, and her involvement throughout was amazing.

To be given a terminal diagnosis at any age is tough, but at just 26 it is something else. After long and tearful discussions with friends and family, Richard's courage and personal drive kicked in yet again. With Mary at his side, as always, life was to be enjoyed. He was not about to waste what remained of his life so he lived it to the full.

July to October 2009

Richard and Mary made donations to leukaemia charities, and utilised the funds from *the Woolley Hat Fund*, in going to various parts of Britain, either by train or by Mary at the wheel of his trusty car. They visited outlying family members, spending time with his mum, sister and both his grandmothers; or simply went to parts of the country they had never been. Postcards were sent from such places as Bowness, Cardiff, the Cavern Club in Liverpool, Paris even, and the cards became a regular part of the postal delivery system.

As the summer went on, Richard experienced shingles and had to have an arm in a sling as all his muscles and nerve ends cried out; and increasingly developed painful ulcers which were indescribable throughout his digestive tract. Those visible in the mouth were so discoloured and large; one could only imagine what Richard was going through. You had to guess, because he never complained about it, preferring to underplay everything. When asked did he ever question the reason for the leukaemia or ask, why me? The instant response typified his character and personality, "No, I don't think that way; instead I think, why not me?" He made us all feel so humble, so often.

In October, it was decided that a special long week-end away would be good for Richard, Mary, Mike, Marion, Emma and Dave to spend some quality time together. We went to Penrith in the Lake District. The weather was generally good and visits were made to see the lakes and places of interest. Richard was by this time unable to eat anything beyond blended food, and it was painful and slow for him to eat more than a few spoonfuls. Whilst there he asked each of us to go to his bedroom, and presented us with a hand-written letter saying what we meant to him and what he expected from us in the future; and gave us a memory box of significant items that would mean something to the recipient. The tears flowed, cuddles and kisses exchanged, sadness was experienced beyond belief – but oh what pride we all felt for such a courageous young man. Our last day there was spent with Richard in a wheelchair in Cockermouth; and then to the sea to fulfil his desire to skim some stones.

Back home again Richard continued to mix with so many friends and family, something which was enormously helpful and meaningful for all involved.

Sadly, Richard's health deteriorated and Mary made the necessary telephone calls to summon key family and friends, including the local priest, to his bedside. Richard and Mary wanted to remain at home; needless to say they had had enough of hospitals. With many around his bed he passed surrounded with love on 22 October 2009.

Words cannot express the loss felt by us all; but the funeral service at the Annunciation Church in Chesterfield (the same one he was married in, with Father McManus too) demonstrated the love we shared for Richard. The young men, family and close friends, carried the coffin in; and the emotion was like a Mexican-wave of tears and sadness uncontrollably sweeping the church. The service was beautifully conducted. On the way to the cemetery the heavens opened and mirrored our feelings. When it came to the actual burial, the sun shone brightly and we all felt this had been arranged specially for us, by Richard himself. The service was accompanied by Richard's favourite song *Don't Look Back into the Sun* by the Libertines.

The Order of Service for his funeral contained a poem written by Richard. Mary discovered the poem inside his journal; the words are deep and meaningful:

Song for a Dead Lover

The church path left behind the crowds
We were together then, but now alone
Our laughter turning back black clouds
She etched a heart in solid stone
Its beat shot dead with an arrow
On a grave with stuffed innards of bone
Life's tightrope, for me, proved too narrow
And I found a cold hole of my own.
Carving deep wounds to leave a trace
The pen tipped rocks trailing dust as she signs
Love weathers death like a hard rock face
As time works on fading our lines.

Omissions

In reading Richard's journal there are certain things which could be deemed unsaid or unfinished. The following may help to complete the gaps.

One key health omission from Richard's journal occurred when he was in the High Dependency Unit during Course 4; and this involved nosebleeds. When a person has no platelets, a nosebleed continues unabated and the extent of blood that can be lost is frightening. Richard's experience of a nosebleed involved lumps and lots of thick blood filling masses of tissues and cloths for over ninety minutes. At a time when fitness, strength and well-being are already low, the effects on the patient can be frightening. Never to be forgotten scenes by those witnessing them. He had more of these later, but thankfully not to the same degree. Pressure bungs fitted by doctors became the only way of stopping these; albeit very uncomfortable for Richard.

Prior to the leukaemia striking, Richard and Mary planned a Mediterranean cruise, incorporating a visit to Rome, for their honeymoon. This had to be cancelled as time went on, as Richard would not have been allowed to go by the doctors, even if he had wanted to. The taking out of holiday insurance was not done initially, so, but for the kindness and understanding of Ocean Village, they would have lost their deposit. Sadly, the same holiday was re-booked in December 2008 when all looked good cure-wise; and the cruise was back on for the following June. Again Ocean Village reimbursed their deposit when the leukaemia returned. Our thanks are extended for their understanding and kindness.

Richard and Mary did in fact get a new roof installed while he was in hospital in 2008. This was paid for by the family, so it did not impact on their wedding budget.

Thankfully, the unhelpfulness of the Nationwide Building Society and the problem with meeting the mortgage payments was overcome by being paid in full – by Richard's Mortgage Protection/Life Policy. Richard jokingly said to Mary when we were talking about this, "I always knew we'd be rich, but I didn't realise I'd have to check out first."

Acknowledgements

Sincere thanks are given to Ann and John, and all their family and friends; yet words alone cannot do justice for all they did to make Richard's life a happy one. The friends that Richard and Mary shared were constant visitors and provided lots of support before and after his death, thank you all so very much.

The staff at the Royal Hallamshire in Sheffield and the Royal Hospital in Chesterfield worked their socks-off to treat and care for Richard. Many of them became like friends and were thought of fondly; our enormous gratitude is extended for all their efforts, professionalism and humanity.

During the treatment Richard received many hundred units of blood and platelet transfusions; and almost stem cells. Heartfelt praise is given to all the anonymous donors who help to keep people alive, and give patients and their families hope too, where, without their generosity there would be none.

Thanks to Seb who created a website for friends and family to post messages and photographs, and this has helped.

What can be said of Mary that is not already self-evident? The love they share is special and will remain unbroken forever. Soul mates without a doubt. She is a treasure.

Conclusion

Richard's key message to all of us for so much of his illness, is simple; love and family. He demonstrated to us how these should be the corner-blocks of life, but sadly we all get caught up in the rat-race or become distracted by insignificant worries and issues. Make time for those you love and demonstrate how important they are to you. Life can change so quickly for any one of us, so do not put it off.

Richard, you are deeply loved and sorely missed, but we have been eternally blessed by you being in our lives.